My Life

Does It Really Matter?

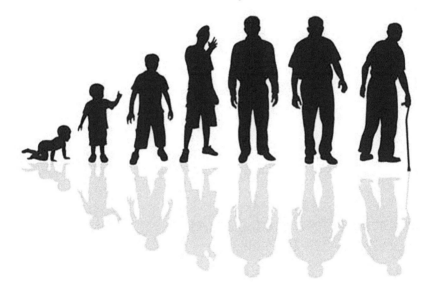

Dick Craig

ISBN 978-1-64299-724-8 (paperback)
ISBN 978-1-64299-725-5 (digital)

Copyright © 2018 by Dick Craig

All rights reserved. No part of this publication may be reproduced, distributed, or transmitted in any form or by any means, including photocopying, recording, or other electronic or mechanical methods without the prior written permission of the publisher. For permission requests, solicit the publisher via the address below.

Christian Faith Publishing, Inc.
832 Park Avenue
Meadville, PA 16335
www.christianfaithpublishing.com

Printed in the United States of America

Contents

Preface 7
My Story 11
    The Lord's Leading and Care 11
    Started Life as a Child 11
Early Days and New Beginnings 13
    School Days—Public School 14
The Little Church on Eramosa Road 18
Guelph Bible Conference Grounds 19
A Growing Family of Craigs 20
    Camp Mini-Yo-We, Mary Lake 20
    Globe and Mail 21
    College Pharmacy 22
High School 23
    Guelph Collegiate Vocational Institute (GCVI) 23
The Call of the Big City (Or Was It the Call to Adventure?) 25
    Toronto 26
The Shoe Business 27
Don 31
Royal Canadian Air Force 33
    Volunteering 34
    Getting Out 36
Back to the Shoe Business 38
    A New Opportunity 39
The Tire Business 41
My Brother Evan 42
Sunday School and My Bride-to-Be 44
    Excitement and Tragedy 45
Bev's Parents and Family 46

Ottawa	48
Growing in Love and in Christ	49
Our Wedding	51
Our First Home	54
Peterborough	55
New Opportunities	57
Stephen	60
Advancement	62
Challenges	63
David and Nancy	65
Advancement	67
Home Ownership	67
Oakwood	68
Carolyn	70
Communication	71
Confidence	74
Moving Again	75
Mark	85
General Crane Industries	86
Excello	91
Janis	93
My Dad	95
Muriel and Bill	97
Multipath Communications	98
Where Do I Go from Here?	101
Niagara	103
Carolyn and Indy	107
Janis and Sean	108
ITP Brampton	110
On the Move Again	111
More of Indy and Carolyn	114
Stephen	114
September 11, 2001	116
Emma	122
More Changes and Challenges	123
Mission Aviation Fellowship of Canada	124

My Brother-in-Law, Bill 136
Maya 137
Jaxson 138
Georgia 139
Niagara (The Second Time!) 140
Charli 142
El Salvador 144
The Last Chapter 149
Insight 153

Preface

Charli is five years old, my youngest granddaughter. On Saturday, we were walking down James Street with Georgia, Charli's older sister, her mom, and her grandmother. Charli and I were walking a little behind. We were headed for the flower shop and to the Vegan donut shop. The donuts were delicious there, but you almost had to take out a mortgage on the house just to buy six of them! Charli and I, walking hand in hand, were talking about God and how He created everything. She said, "Grandpa, where did God come from?" I answered that God was always there, from the very beginning. She said, "But, Grandpa, who made God?" What an intriguing question!

A few years ago, my good friend, Barry, invited me to a meeting. The group would meet monthly and called themselves IdeaShare. Many who attended were either entrepreneurs or self-employed business people. For the most part, they were all intellectuals. (Not sure why I was invited.) The idea was to come with an idea, something that would perhaps intrigue the others or, at least, cause dialogue. I wondered what idea I could bring. So, when it was my turn, I remember asking them to consider three questions:

1. Where did you come from?
2. Why are you here?
3. Where are you going?

No one spoke. Perhaps, after all these years, each one is still considering the questions and the answers for themselves.

My purpose in writing this book is multifaceted: to share my life memories with my family and friends, to challenge whoever picks up this book to consider my three questions for themselves, and to come to realize that the God of heaven exists and is indeed faithful and trustworthy and that He loves them with an incredible love. My greatest desire is that my total family including nephews, nieces, and their children would give their hearts and lives to Him. I'll guarantee that in the long run, it will be without regret.

You can "take that one to the bank"!

Yesterday was Sunday! After Pastor Larry spoke so clearly on Joseph's life and God caring and His provision through it all, we sang this song written by Fanny J. Crosby, written more than two hundred years ago!

> All the way my Savior leads me,
> What have I to ask beside?
> Can I doubt His tender mercy,
> Who through life has been my Guide?
> Heav'nly peace, divinest comfort,
> Here by faith in Him to dwell!
> For I know, whate'er befall me,
> Jesus doeth all things well;
> For I know, whate'er befall me,
> Jesus doeth all things well.
> All the way my Savior leads me,
> Cheers each winding path I tread,
> Gives me grace for every trial,
> Feeds me with the living Bread.
> Though my weary steps may falter
> And my soul athirst may be,
> Gushing from the Rock before me,
> Lo! A spring of joy I see;
> Gushing from the Rock before me,
> Lo! A spring of joy I see.
> All the way my Savior leads me,
> Oh, the fullness of His love!
> Perfect rest to me is promised
> In my Father's house above.

> When my spirit, clothed immortal,
> Wings its flight to realms of day
> This my song through endless ages:
> Jesus led me all the way;
> This my song through endless ages:
> Jesus led me all the way.

This song, these words are my testimony. I can look back now and see God's hand in my life.

Many years ago, Christian artist, Steve Green wrote a song that sticks in my memory and outlines my intention and, I believe, my responsibility for writing this book. When I'm gone, what footprints, what signposts will I leave that will inspire others, especially my family, to place their complete trust in the Savior whom I love! My desire, above all else, is to bring joy to the heart of God; however, He allows me to do that!

> We're pilgrims on the journey of the narrow road,
> and those who've gone before us line the way.
> cheering on the faithful, encouraging the weary,
> their lives a stirring testament to God's sustaining grace.
>
> Surrounded by so great a cloud of witnesses,
> let us run the race not only for the prize,
> but as those who've gone before us, let us leave
> to those behind us, the heritage of faithfulness
> passed on thru godly lives.
> O may all who come behind us find us faithful,
> may the fire of our devotion light their way.
> may the footprints that we leave, lead them to believe,
> and the lives we live inspire them to obey.
> O may all who come behind us find us faithful.

DICK CRAIG

After all our hopes and dreams have come and gone,
and our children sift thru all we've left behind,
may the clues that they discover, and the memories they uncover,
become the light that leads them, to the road we each must find.

O may all who come behind us find us faithful,
may the fire of our devotion light their way.
may the footprints that we leave, lead them to believe,
and the lives we live inspire them to obey.
O may all who come behind us find us faithful.

My Story

The Lord's Leading and Care

We all have a story! A very personal story. It's our story. It's nobody else's. We're the only one who has lived our story. It's personal! It's important! It's our "DNA." Our story is full of twists and turns, experiences, adventures, heartaches, disappointments, longings, and joy and sadness. They're all in our memory, some at the forefront of our minds, many distant, like whiffs of smoke that appear suddenly in an azure sky, staying for a time, and then disappearing again. As we look back, we can feel them, remember them, and they often guide our thoughts connecting them with other thoughts and memories! We reminisce, sometimes causing us to be thrilled or discouraged or other emotions that come to the surface. We humans are complex. It's the way God made us. We're fearfully and wonderfully made—made in God's image, made in His likeness, made for His pleasure, made for His glory alone!

Started Life as a Child

Here's my story! I started life as a child! I heard a comedian say that once and never forgot it! But it's true, isn't it? We all start out that way! There's no other way to start! It reminds what the Bible states, how when someone is "born again" they require the "sincere milk of the word." That's how a newborn starts out. That's how I started out. I just don't remember that part. I was born on April 3, 1940, to my parents, Ruth and Trevor Craig. I was born in Paris, Ontario, about sixteen kilometers northwest of Brantford, Ontario, where Mother and Dad lived with my two older brothers, David and

James. Dad was a beekeeper along with his father, and my mother was already a busy mom, David being just two years and four months old and James eleven months younger. Little did any of us know that in sixteen years, there would be eleven of us kids. I remember when the matter of our large family came up at the dinner table, my father would often quote from the passage in Psalm 127. He'd tell us with a smile: "Happy is the man whose quiver is full of them!"

The scripture states:

Lo, children are an heritage of the LORD: and the fruit of the womb is his reward. As arrows are in the hand of a mighty man; so are children of the youth. Happy is the man that hath his quiver full of them: they shall not be ashamed, but they shall speak with the enemies in the gate. (Psalm 127:3–5, KJV)

My dad and mother loved their large family and truly believed that they were blessed beyond measure. And they were!

Early Days and New Beginnings

I have just a few memories from those Brantford days, living on Grand Avenue next to the "County Barns." My Uncle Sam worked there and lived with us. There was a "stile" over the fence between properties, and my older brothers and I would climb the stile steps to the top of the wire fence with Uncle Sam's lunch and call, "Uncle Sam, here's your lunch." He would come out of the county barn and take it from us with a smile and a thank you! Great memories! My Great Aunt Ethel, Dad's Aunt, lived just down the street from us in a small bungalow surrounded by trees and grapevines. We often walked with Dad to visit her. My sister, Muriel, was born in 1941. That made four of us. And then in 1943, the day after April fools, Mom gave birth to Evan, her fourth son and, obviously, my third brother. At least I wasn't the baby of the family any longer! In 1944, Sylvia came along.

The score is boys, 4, while girls, 2. The girls are still outnumbered, two to four!

Our dad, Trevor, had graduated from Ontario Agriculture College in apiculture (beekeeping) in 1936, in Guelph, Ontario; and in 1945, he received an opportunity to teach apiculture at the Guelph college. So, in the summer of that year, Dad and Mom packed up the six kids, all the beekeeping equipment, and our belongings and followed the moving truck to an old red-brick house on the outskirts of Guelph. I remember the year and the move! The kids were excited. We all were! What an adventure! Even though I was only five, that year is still fresh in my memory. I remember it for two reasons. I would start school in September, and it was the end of World War II. I distinctly remember many airplanes flying over our house in early September, as the RCAF celebrated this historic event. David, James, and I were mesmerized, hearing the engines, watching the airplanes swoop and dive overhead, waving their wings, even though we didn't understand what it all meant.

School Days—Public School

Macdonald Consolidated School was our new world, at least for Dave, James, and myself. I had never gone to school before and so the adventure continued. This was "old hat" for my older brothers. They'd already attended school in Brantford, but it was all new to me. Our school was a stately building with two floors and six or seven classrooms, almost colonial in appearance. It was surrounded by a neatly groomed campus and several trees. Macdonald Consolidated stood adjacent to the Ontario Agriculture College, which sprawled for a mile or so to the east. That's where our dad taught beekeeping to college students. To get to our school, we walked west on College Avenue, a gravel road, down the hill through "skunk hollow" (we named it that because of the many skunks that lived in the creek there and you could smell them as we walked by on the road), then up the college hill, past the college student dining hall and "Mac," the lady's college, to our public school on the northwest campus. It was about a quarter of a mile, but in the winter, it seemed a lot farther. We used to go home at noon for lunch. Sometimes the "Baker" (we called the bread man that, because he delivered bread and cakes to our house by horse-drawn wagon) was parked by our house, feeding his horse, just about the time we were heading back to school. I remember climbing onto his wagon and asking him if he had any stale cookies. He'd often open a fresh pack and gave us "urchins" a cookie; then he would unhitch the food bag from his horse and give us a ride back to school. Those were the good old days!

I have many memories of public school days! In early 1947, my brother Paul was born. I was seven years old and I remember mother coming home from the hospital with baby Paul and placing him (just for fun) in Muriel's doll buggy, and he just fit! Paul made seven of us. Two years later, in June of 1949, Fred was born! Wow, this was getting out of hand! Eight kids! And our parents weren't finished yet.

We didn't know it, nobody knew it, but there were three more to come! "Children are a blessing from the Lord and my father's 'quiver' was getting mighty full!"

I remember the kids at school used to taunt us about our big family. I recall how they used disparaging and bullying remarks about my dad and mom. These really did hurt, but my siblings and I were not ashamed. We were proud of our big family. We had a wonderful mother and father. They cared for us and loved us. We didn't even think about how poor we were in terms of material things. Our parents showed us through their example that we were extremely rich in the things that mattered and so very valuable to them and to the Lord whom they loved.

Public school was a challenge for me, especially grade three! There were about thirty-five students who were seated according to their ability by Mrs. Tolten's standards. She was a disciplinarian, to be sure, and I was a bit of a rebel. You see, I had two older brothers to keep up to. Mrs. Tolten's favorites were student monitors. These (special) students sat in the first three or four seats of the first row because their "interest marks" were the best. I was never assigned to be a monitor by Mrs. Tolten. Every grade three and four student in her classroom had his or her name on her blackboard and gained "interest marks" for good behavior, good marks on assignments, and generally being attentive students. That didn't particularly fit me, you see. I was "cool" (or whatever they called us back in those days), so my marks on the board allowed me, most often, to sit in the very back seat of row three. By the way, I failed grade three the first time! Got first class honors the second time around! It only took me two years to do it!

Explaining all this to my parents was a challenge, of course; they seemed to take my teacher's position over mine, especially when I brought my report card for the needed parent signature. My father was also in the "education business." He applied "the board of education to the seat of learning." I remember my dad saying that this punishment hurt him more than it hurt me. I always had trouble understanding that statement! Looking back, I deserved it, but at the time I had a different opinion. That "board" hurt!

Bill was a tough guy. He was about my age and in my class. He could speak like Donald Duck! We called him "Digger," but he was known as "Do or Die, Dare Devil, Digger Dawson, Donald Duck." That's what he liked to be called, especially by his peers and us underlings. He ran things, he and his friend David. Sometimes the two of them would follow me partway home after school, taunting me about our family or our circumstances. I remember one time, they grabbed my loose-leaf three-ring binder with my notes and homework, opened it, made a pathway with the papers, and then they both walked on top of them on the grass of the campus. I was in tears when I arrived home! I often wonder what happened to "Digger" and David!

In spite of those early challenges and opposition, there were especially good happenings along the way. One thing that stands out is when I was nine years old. My mother and dad loved the Lord and spoke of Him often in our home. We learned so much from them about Jesus' love for each of us and how we needed to trust Him and personally give our lives to Him. We were never pressured! My mother would often speak to us kids lovingly about the Lord as she prepared food in the kitchen or rolled pastry for pies at the kitchen table. (She sometimes made six or seven pies at a time; they never lasted long in our house!) Dad would open his Bible at the table after supper and share a devotion. His favorite passage was Proverbs 3:5–6:

Trust in the LORD with all thine heart; and lean not unto thine own understanding.

In all thy ways acknowledge him, and he shall direct thy paths.

This was the way he and mom lived. This was their motto, and this was the foundation they were laying for their children.

After school during the fall, winter, and spring, there was a Good News Club held in the school basement once a week for any student who wished to attend. My parents encouraged us all to attend. I remember it was led by two of the lady teachers from our school (but can't remember their names). These ladies were fine Christians. They taught us Bible stories, and we sang choruses and played fun games. It was a great break from school. One day I remember being intrigued by one of the Bible stories, and there was a stirring in my heart. Even as a nine-year-old, I sensed that there was something missing in my life. After, I asked one of the teachers to help me to understand. She was so gentle and kind, and she spoke to me and explained how I might accept Jesus into my life. She and I prayed, and that day, I received Jesus as my Lord and Savior. I raced home, over the school campus, past the college dining hall, down the hill through "skunk hollow" up the other side past the Cutten Fields Golf Club to our red-brick house calling, as loud as I could, "Mom, Dad, I'm saved!" Although there have been many "hills and valleys" in my Christian walk since that day, there is no doubt in my heart and mind that my decision that day was the beginning of my walk with Christ. At this writing, that was sixty-eight years ago. As I look back, there is an immense joy and thankfulness that fills and thrills my being and it doesn't go away! The scripture tells us that when we receive Christ, we are given the gift of God's Holy Spirit. He makes His home in us. He permanently lives in everyone who places his or her trust in Christ. I will guarantee you that this is true!

The Little Church on Eramosa Road

Every Sunday morning, our growing family would pile into the old Buick station wagon and head to Eramosa Gospel Hall, just north of where we lived, maybe three or four miles away, close to the city center. There were two services on Sunday morning, Breaking of Bread (Communion) at nine o'clock and family Bible hour at eleven o'clock. At three o'clock to four o'clock in the afternoon was Sunday school for all ages. We returned again at 7:00 p.m., for the "gospel meeting." Sunday was a day full of church. We didn't call it "church" though! The church was the people, not the building. We called it "the chapel" or "the gospel hall." We never went to "church." We were the "church."

This was a Plymouth Brethren Gospel Hall, undenominational to be sure! We held two New Testament teachings, the elders being in charge. There was no pastor or minister, only men of God to lead worship and to preach and teach. I must say, these leaders, for the most part, knew their Bibles well. They taught, encouraged, and trained young men of the assembly to study the scriptures and occasionally gave them opportunity to speak from the platform. The women were silent! But it was a good community. We felt secure there and loved by many! I remember trooping into "Breaking of Bread" service, always a few minutes late, with all the family, Dad and Mother at the front of the line followed by David, then James, and so on, like "steps going down." They usually saved the first two rows for "the Craig army." I felt we were always viewed as a bit of a "spectacle." But these were good days for us. They were "foundational."

Guelph Bible Conference Grounds

Every year, from the first of July until the end of August, the elders closed the Gospel Hall and the whole congregation moved to the Guelph Bible Conference Grounds. This was a big deal, especially for the Craig children. We were free for the summer, sort of! The Grounds were really in the middle of the city but very remote in that they were surrounded by trees, not visible at all from the road. For us kids, it was like being in a different world. Brethren people came to the conference from all over North America, even as far away as Texas. It was like a summer Christian Camp for all ages. The grounds had been the McAlister farm in the 1930s and was gifted to the Christian Assemblies for a conference center. There was a large farm house on the property called Century Lodge. In those days, this old house doubled as an inn with accommodations and a dining hall. The property, which covered approximately fifteen to twenty acres, included ten or so small log cabins for families and staff. We loved this place! And, for my brothers and me, there were girls, from all over! My future wife, Beverley (although I didn't know it at the time), came from Windsor with her two sisters. This Conference stuff was a big deal. There were many excellent Bible teachers that came. I remember one especially, whose name was Alfred P. Gibbs, APG., for short! He called himself that! He told us the APG really meant "a perfect gentleman." I'm not sure he was "a perfect gentleman." I don't remember any of his Bible teaching, but, boy, I remember that APG could really play table tennis! He beat everyone. He was my "Ping-Pong" champion! Growing up, our family spent every summer at "The Grounds." Such fond memories!

A Growing Family of Craigs

In July 1951, Bill Saunders Craig was born into our ever-growing family. Then in late 1952, Mark Alexander Craig came into the world. That made ten of us! Two years later, in November 1954, Ian Clement Craig appeared. (I thought my parents were going to run out of names. After all, we had two names each!) Ian made it eleven! And that was it. Mother and Dad never quite made the dozen! And even though there were lots of us, we always felt loved and secure. We never knew we were poor! We never felt it, because we weren't, not in the things that mattered!

Camp Mini-Yo-We, Mary Lake

Camp Mini-Yo-We was a new Christian Camp located on Mary Lake near Huntsville, Ontario. Mini-Yo-We is an Indian name meaning "Camp of Living Waters." The camp was situated in a beautiful Muskoka setting surrounded by woods; it was the perfect spot! For the Craig boys, to attend, two weeks at camp, was a distant dream; our parents would never be able to afford it. It was beyond our imagination; still, we could dream.

The elders at Eramosa Road Gospel Hall really had the Craig family at heart. After all, there were so many of us! The church leaders had a fund set aside to help send kids to camp. Then, seemingly "out of the blue," my oldest brother, David, was sent by the elders. Dad drove him there, and James and I got to go along for the ride. Mom packed our lunch and David's suitcase, our first overnight adventure ever! It was fabulous. We slept overnight on the floor of an old house on the camp property. Two years later, they sent me to camp. It was a dream come true! The church elders sent me again, two years later!

The experiences for me at Camp Mini-Yo-We were life-changing. Successful camping experiences require three things: dry and safe accommodations, good food, and a well-planned and well-executed program. All three were well met! The leadership was amazing! We all had nicknames, mine was "Stretch." I don't know why, as I was one of the short ones. Each night we all gathered at "Campfire Point." It was a jut of land right on the edge of the water with a huge bonfire between us campers and the water. We sat on rows of half-buried logs stretched across the clearing and tiered behind us. As we looked out on the sunset, we'd sing choruses at the top of our voices, then suddenly stop and listen to the echo from across the lake. It was magical! We were challenged by amazing leaders, who shared Christ's love. We listened attentively as boys and leaders shared their testimonies, how God had worked in their lives. It was such a great and memorable time for all of us. We made great friends with other boys and established real bonds with our cabin leaders. Then, it was back to our cabin for snacks, devotions, and "lights out." After the first night, we were exhausted! So many good and memorable experiences. A few years later, I had the privilege of going to Mini-Yo-We as cabin leader! Even after all these years, I am still so grateful to those folks from Eramosa Road Gospel Hall who underwrote the cost to send me to camp. It really did change my life and helped me to begin to walk the path that I travel even now. I guess I should really say, "To God be the glory," and I do say that!

Globe and Mail

David, James, and I had a Globe and Mail route. In order to get all the newspapers delivered and get to school on time, we needed to get up at 6:00 a.m. Good old Dad, he'd wake us up and encourage us to get ready and be on our way. We had to walk to the administration building at the college (about a quarter of a mile) where the bundle of papers was waiting. We'd fold them all, and we were on our way. My brothers had split the route into three. At the end of each week, we would collect from our customers. We earned a few cents each week for delivery plus sometimes a quarter or two in tips. At Christmas time, the tips were much better! This was our first business venture! I think I was ten years old at the time!

College Pharmacy

When I was in grade six, I got an after-school job at the College Pharmacy, across Gordon Street from our school. Jake and John were the owners and my bosses. My job was to deliver "phoned in" orders with my bicycle. I can't remember exactly, but I think John paid me two dollars a week. I worked every day after school from 4:00 until 6:00. If there wasn't anything to deliver, I'd sweep the floor and looked after the garbage. That was my job! Sometimes, when I got it for free, I had ice cream at the lunch counter which was part of the drugstore. I loved those days! I remember one time I was in the back room of the store bundling up the garbage to take out the back door to the garbage can. The back door was old with a glass window, and as I reached for the door, the glass window fell out on my left arm, cutting a deep gash just above my wrist. Fortunately, Jake, the pharmacist, was right there and knew what to do. I still bear the mark though! Rough job that!

High School

I finally graduated from Macdonald Consolidated Public School. I was fourteen years old. I really felt I was quite mature and I had all this cool business experience, working at the drugstore and delivering the Globe and Mail. Besides, I had worked for my dad for the last couple of summers (along with my brothers) extracting honey and filling pails in his "honey house" plus sold honey door-to-door and at the Guelph market. The honey house, by the way, was the small white barn at the back end of our property where my father had all his beekeeping apparatus including extractors, honey strainer equipment, holding tanks for pure honey, plus pails, lids, etc. Anyway, I was well on my way to a successful business career; it's just that school was in the way. By the way, I graduated from grade eight with first class honors; my marks tied with three other guys.

Guelph Collegiate Vocational Institute (GCVI)

Well, in September I got to high school, grade nine, and thought, "What a waste of time!" Here I am stuck when I could be out making my fortune. When I started GCVI, I got an "after school" job for Thursday, Friday, and all day Saturday. The store was in a higher-grade shoe store called Scott Shoes, right on the main street of Guelph. Mr. Scott taught me how to fit and sell quality and corrective shoes. I enjoyed the work immensely and loved the people, even the difficult customers. Mr. Scott paid me $12.00 per week. I paid my mom $5.00 weekly for board and bought my own clothes and covered my expenses with the rest.

GCVI was different from public school. The guys there were really a wild bunch, at least the guys I knew. They told me that GCVI stood for Guelph's Collection of Vicious Idiots, and I felt I was one of them. My friend, Bill, and I would take off after last class of the day and head two or three blocks to the YMCA where we played "Snooker and Boston" on the pool table. Bill taught me how to play, and over time I became pretty good. I also took up smoking. At first, I hated it, but I wanted to be like the other "cool guys," so I persisted. I got "good" at that too! I smoked from age fourteen until I was about twenty. I used to lie to my parents that I never smoked, but they could smell it on my clothes. Still, they loved me anyway! I'm certainly not very proud of this part of my life! As I improved at billiards, I needed more competition, so I often headed down to the local "pool hall" on the main street. The guys who "hung out" there were older and much more experienced. I improved even more! My father found out and barred me from going there. I disobeyed him a time or two but mostly stayed away. I always said that being a "pool shark" was the sign of "an ill-spent youth!"

Those early high school day relationships did nothing for me, because I was a rebel and independent and wanted to live my own life. I was far from my Christian roots, from my confession of faith at the age of nine. I know my parents were worried and prayed for me daily, but I was headstrong and wanted to live my own life and make my own way.

The Call of the Big City
(Or Was It the Call to Adventure?)

In spite of myself, I graduated grade nine in June and moved on to grade ten. Starting grade ten was a pain. School was not for me! I needed my freedom to find my own way. I needed to make money. My parents encouraged me to stay in school, to apply myself, but I'd made up my mind. I quit! I was barely sixteen. I applied for a job at Hammond Electric on Wellington Street, where they designed and built transformers. I became a coil winder! I worked hard sitting at this little winding machine, attaching leads to thin copper wire, and then winding the coils to the right size with different sizes of copper wire. Man, this was boring work, but I got paid, I was earning money. Mother and Dad were not happy, neither was I, really! I worked at Hammond for three months and for Ernie Scott at the shoe store on the weekends.

The "shoe business" was much more intriguing for me and much more satisfying! I asked Mr. Scott if he would hire me full-time, but he had a full-time employee and not able to take on a second one. I'm sure he would have if he could! However, he knew a man in Toronto, a Mr. Pollock who owned forty-three shoe stores in Toronto and surrounding region. He told me he would be pleased to arrange a meeting and an interview with Mr. Pollock and even write a letter of recommendation for me. That was if I could get to Toronto on my own. Wow! Here was my chance!

I was only sixteen, but I was an adventurer at heart. Nothing was impossible. Somehow, in my heart, I was convinced that Mr. Pollock would hire me. In the next few days, I was in downtown Toronto, sitting in Mr. Pollock's office, letter in hand. I can't now remember exactly how I got there. Toronto was fifty or so miles from Guelph. I might have traveled by Greyhound or hitch-hiked but don't remember exactly! But I got there! I had no fear! I liked Mr. Pollock immediately, and he seemed to like me. He hired me to work in a small store on Kingston Road in Scarborough. I believe the manager's name was Cliff. Some names escape me now, since that was in 1956, about fifty-seven years ago. I had no idea where I would live or how I would get to my new job, and my parents did not know I even had a job there. I just figured it would work out. After all, God would provide, somehow! Our mother and dad had instilled this principle in all the kids! I just wasn't sure how, when, why, or even how Mother and Dad would even react. Their third son was leaving the nest!

Toronto

My job in Toronto was to begin in one week. Even though they had many misgivings, Mother and Dad drove me along with my suitcase. (I remember it was a worn brown leather folding case, like a valise, that my father had used during his college days.) It carried most of my "earthly possessions," to the YMCA in downtown Toronto. As I look back now, I'm reminded of the story of the prodigal son in Luke 11, not because I asked my father to divide my inheritance or give me my share (I'm sure there would have been very little) or not to live lavishly or wastefully but to have an adventure and to make my fortune. I was so headstrong and so determined! Perhaps that was the intention of the prodigal in the beginning. But the core of it all, I believe, was it was breaking my father's and my mother's heart, just as the prodigal did in Luke 11. I know that his mother is not mentioned in scripture, but my guess is that it was true. My dad and mother were really "as one!" God in His wisdom and grace and love had "welded" them together, and I'm sure, at the moment they let me off in Toronto, their hearts were breaking. I wonder what it was like, on their drive home.

The Shoe Business

It was Saturday and my new job at Pollocks would begin the following Monday, in just two days. I needed to find a place to live, fast! I found a newspaper with want ads and looked under "Accommodations, Room and Board." There were several offered in Toronto's east end, and after a few calls, I found something that sounded affordable. My salary was thirty dollars weekly, and I believe the board amount was twenty dollars per week including all meals. My landlady packed me a lunch; she and her husband were so very kind to me; maybe they felt sorry for me. She also did my laundry and provided snacks! My prayers had been answered, and it was only about a twenty-minute streetcar ride to and from work. The ten dollars leftover was tight, considering streetcar fare and all, but I made it work. I was now in the "big-time," a good job, and my independence. What more could I ask for. I was on my way to making my fortune! I had no idea what lay ahead! I enjoyed working with Cliff who'd been managing the Kingston Road store for a long time. His clientele loved him. He taught me how to deal with people. It was great training! For a time, I was content, sort of! I wondered what was next and wanted a new challenge. Cliff saw that, and a few months later, I had the opportunity to move to a busier store at Coxwell and Danforth. This store was managed by an Englishman. My new job was a long way from my digs, so I found a new boarding place at Jarvis and Dundas. At that time Jarvis Street was known as the "red light" district. It didn't deter me! I was sixteen, almost seventeen, fearless and confident.

I lived in a boarding house on Dundas Street close to Jarvis, with four or five other men. We each had our own room. This was an old house, kind of decrepit, and situated right on the edge of Dundas Street close to the intersection. The street car stop was right out front. Our landlord was a phenomenal cook and made us wonderful meals at suppertime, beginning with homemade soup, then a plate piled high with roast beef, mashed potatoes with gravy, and loads of vegetables. A feast every day! As I recall, I had worked at the Coxwell store for only a short time, perhaps two or three months, when an opportunity came up at a larger, new store at Cloverdale Mall in Toronto's west end. I was now seventeen and had all this experience "under my belt." I was ready for the big move. I would be assistant manager under Lorne, the store manager, at Cloverdale Mall! Lorne was rated one of the top managers in the whole Pollock chain. Wow! What an opportunity. I would be earning thirty-five dollars a week. I just had to find a new place to live.

There is a definite "thread" that winds its way through my life as I look back. It seems to me, and I believe it to be true, that God had His hand on me and still does! As I look back today, I'm reminded of the story of the man who confronted God, saying that he had been deserted and had to tread his path alone. God pointed out his footprints in the sand, and in many places, there were two sets. But in other places during lonely and difficult times, there was only one set. The man pointed this out to God, that on these occasions, he walked alone. But God said to him, "No, my son, where there are only one set of footprints, I was carrying you."

There were people along the way that, I believe, were strategically placed to guide me and protect me, even from myself, at times. For the most part, these were just ordinary people. I know I was not living as a Christian during those early days, but there was a definite sense of right and wrong there, deep in my spirit. These principles and values were constantly demonstrated to each of us kids by our mother and dad from the first day of our lives. These became indelibly part of our DNA. But over all of this was and is the amazing "umbrella" of God's incredible love. My main purpose in sharing "my adventures" is to tell you and show you and demonstrate to you that this same wonderful love is extended to you and to anyone. You and I are of incredible value to God Himself! He crafted you and He crafted me in His own image, in His own likeness, and He desires us to trust Him more than anything else, even more than life itself!

Well, Cloverdale Mall and my job as assistant manager of Pollock Shoes, to me, was the "big-time!" I had arrived, and I was only seventeen. I had life around the throat, and I was on my way! I found a place to stay on Silverhill Drive, Etobicoke, within walking distance of my new job. The elderly couple who owned the bungalow were wonderful. The weekly cost was affordable, and I got my laundry done and a lunch "packed." Just down the street lived the "Green family." I met Don Green, a guy about my age, soon after I moved there. Little did I know it, but the whole Green family would become a significant part of my life.

During my time at Cloverdale, the first time that is, I learned a great deal about managing. (I worked there, left for a while, and then returned; that part will come later.) My manager was experienced and taught me well. He would often leave me in charge and return one or two hours later. He had other interests at Cloverdale! I often ran the store alone except on weekends when a couple of part-time staff worked. I was the boss when Lorne wasn't there. Man, I was cool! Everything didn't always run smoothly, though. One incident stands out clearly in my mind.

Each night before closing, we removed the cash from the "till," placed it in a cloth bag, and hid it in a random shoe box behind one of the partitions where the inventory was kept. Lorne and I knew the designated box. No one else did. We were sworn to secrecy. In the morning, we would retrieve the cash, place it back in the cash register, and begin the day. This was our routine! Sometimes, during busy season, we'd remove excess cash during the day and hide it in our predetermined place. We were very careful about this! On one of those occasions, when we were busy, I took my break and left the store for lunch. Lorne was away, I believe, and I and other staff were working the evening shift. When I returned, the hidden money was gone. It was reported at once, and the police arrived on the scene. We were all interviewed, but for some reason, I was "centered out." I was taken to the detective's car and grilled by two burly officers who were insistent that I had taken the money and that all I needed to do was confess, return it, and all would be forgiven. I had no clue who had taken it, but it wasn't me. After what seemed like hours, they let me out of the car and allowed me to return to the store. What an experience to be accused, threatened, and made to feel guilty. The money and the thief were never found.

Don

My friendship with Don, my neighbor down the street, developed and grew. We discovered that we both liked fishing and pool. Don worked at a book-binding company operating a "gluing" machine. Don introduced me to his mom whom we both affectionately called Ma and his dad who he'd nicknamed Charly. "Charly's" real name was Norm. Marylou was Don's younger sister. We all got along famously right from the start! I was accepted as one of the family. We did crazy things together like giving their dog, "Trixie," toffee and then holding his jaws together and then letting him go, just to see if he had trouble opening his mouth. The poor dog would run around the house shaking his head until he was able to open his mouth and eat the candy and then he'd come back for more. One day Don brought a pet monkey home to show "Ma." She hated monkeys! The monkey was a pet of one of the people Don worked with at the book-binding plant. Don perched the monkey on his mother's shoulder, and it proceeded to totally relieve himself all down Ma's back. Some days, in winter, Don and I would coax Ma to come to the front door, push her outside, and lock her out in the cold, not for long, of course. We were always in trouble, but she was always so good-natured. This was all in fun, of course. I learned to love Ma and Charly very quickly. I was like their second son!

The Greens had a summer cottage in Bowmanville, Ontario, a good hour and half from where we lived in Etobicoke. Often, I was invited to go along with them for the weekend. We would all travel together in Charly's car, piled high with people, suitcases, and food. There was Ma, Charly, Marylou, Don, and me and the dog, of course! The trip down and back and the weekend itself were hilarious. Don and I and Trixie fished and hiked along the water and up through the reeds. We caught pike; at least Don caught pike! I don't ever remember catching anything but sunken logs and branches and maybe the odd rubber boot but never fish, at least of any size. But we had fun! These were great days and great memories!

Don and I talked about everything, our dreams, girls (of course), fishing, etc. He often told me about the forty-two-inch pike that he caught in the reeds not far from the Bowmanville cottage; he was so proud of that one! I could only talk about the ones that got away! I shared my life with Don. I told him of my faith in God and how our parents had taught us from the scriptures about giving our lives to Christ and that I had done that as a young boy. I emphasized to him that he should consider doing that for himself. Of course, my life example at that time was not the best, and Don just took what I said "with a grain of salt."

Royal Canadian Air Force

Don and I talked about quitting our jobs and joining the RCAF together and seeing the world. We dreamed about that "adventure" until one day, it became a reality. Together, we went down to the local recruitment office and "signed up," took the required medical examination, and waited excitedly to be accepted! It took a while! Finally, the official notification came in the mail. Don was rejected because he was underweight, but I was accepted! Both of us were devastated, but I couldn't back out. I was officially committed for five years. A month or so later, I was on a train heading to the RCAF boot camp in Saint Jean, Quebec, without my best buddy! I was eighteen! Wow, the twists and turns of life are really something, especially when they're self-inflicted!

Well, being the adventurer that I was (and still am, by the way), I made the best of it! Life was tough at boot camp, and I wasn't used to rules. We slept in a barracks with about eighteen other guys, guys as green as I was! That was an experience! Lights out at 10:00 p.m., rising time 5:00 a.m. (whether you liked it or not), mess hall at five thirty, fully dressed. Back to the barracks before 7:00 a.m., beds made, and shoes spit-shined so that the corporal could see his face in them. And there we stood, dressed in full uniform, at full attention at the foot of our beds. We were ready for inspection, not a hair out of place nor a snicker on a face.

The mess hall experiences stand out in my mind. At each meal we would line up, tray in hand, and move quickly along the front of the serving table. Cooks/servers, each standing in front of a pot of "something" with serving spoon raised (almost like a weapon), were ready to plop whatever it was on your plate. You needed to be on "high alert" during this process! An unsuspecting airman might receive a piece of chocolate cake and then a spoonful of gravy over it. These servers enjoyed doing this, especially with the unsuspecting new arrivals. You just had to be on guard at all times!

Every day, we marched for many hours it seemed and dressed in full gear with rifles battle ready! (It's a blessing the rifles weren't loaded.) In the beginning, most of us had two left feet and sounded almost like a herd of stumbling buffalo as we stomped down the pavilion, trying desperately to keep in line. Our corporal was a tough drill noncommissioned officer (NCO). No nonsense! He was tough as nails! We developed a consuming hatred for the man; he was unreasonable as far as we were concerned. When he commanded "halt," we were to slam our left foot down as hard as we could on the concrete, in total unison, one sound. We repeated it again and again, trying to make the sound louder each time. The corporal, our drill NCO, suggested that we should consider that his face was under our left foot every time we came to a halt. The sound increased dramatically! The days were long and often tense, but we were all improving, and after several weeks, we became a precision marching unit.

On special "march past" days, our squad and the other squads would, in turn, march sharply past the commanding officer and his entourage, rifles on our shoulders, our eyes averted left, and, in single motion, raise our right hands in salute. This was done with precision and with great deal of pride! We were finally a "fighting unit," ready for battle! I believe Corporal Hollins breathed a sigh of relief after we had completed the parade march without error. After all, his reputation was on the line. We wouldn't dare let the corporal down. That is if we valued our lives at all!

Volunteering

There are two instances that stand out in my memory during my twelve weeks in St. Jean Quebec, things that were dramatic, at least for me! One such instance occurred within two or three weeks after my arrival. Our squad was just getting to know Corporal Hollins. One morning during marching, he called a halt and commanded us to "stand easy." He had an announcement to make. He said he was looking for volunteers to give blood for the blood bank that was scheduled for the following morning and he had decided that the whole squad would be volunteers, all of us, no exceptions. Probably all thirty-three of us had never given blood before in our lives! But he said we would be rewarded afterward, with a glass of orange juice and donuts! Wow!

The next morning, we all arrived, on time of course, for this "volunteer project!" One by one we were escorted into a cubicle and onto a narrow cot covered with a white sheet. The medical personnel proceeded to insert the needle and draw the blood. After the initial shock wore off, it wasn't all that bad. We were brave guys, part of a fighting unit! After the procedure was done, we were given the prize, the juice and donuts. I was famished, and I drank and ate it fast. I felt light-headed and stood up to leave. That's the last thing I remember until I woke up, lying on the cold linoleum floor and staring at two very shiny black boots right at my head. I blearily looked up into the smiling face of Corporal Hollins. He looked down at me from his height and said, "Craig, what are you doing down there?"

The other incident that stands out in my mind was another volunteer arrangement. But this time it was truly volunteer! We were given the opportunity, as individuals, to be involved in an "experiment," like a military medical trial of sorts. The details are foggy in my mind, but I'll try to remember as much as I can.

Apparently, the Canadian armed forces medical division had developed a serum to combat mustard gas and they needed "guinea pigs" to test this on. Mustard gas was a poisonous gas used during World War I. This dangerous gas, when released on the enemy, attacked the eyes, skin, and respiratory system, sometimes blinding the troops, often making them violently ill, thus rendering them helpless and at the mercy of the enemy. This opportunity was a bit scary for us, even though, for the most part, we were "tough guys." The prize for us was three days' leave with extra pay. Quite of few of us said we were in, including me! I wasn't going to be left behind. After all, three days' off with extra pay was a big deal. The next morning the guys and I arrived at the special clinic within the compound, a bit apprehensive to say the least. We were not sure where this would lead! There were a few curtained off areas in the room; each containing a strange-looking plywood apparatus propped vertically on the floor with what looked like a two by four strut hinged to the underside of the one-inch plywood sheet. On the face of the sheet, about a third of the way down, was an attached leather shoulder and chest harness, almost like one you would see on a parachute. We weren't sure what was coming! We were called in three or four at a time into different makeshift curtained rooms where they attached the harness to each of us as we stood with our backs to the vertical board. We were then given a couple of pills in a little paper cup to swallow with water. This was an antidote to mustard gas. Then the gas was applied, I don't remember how. I do remember the medical scientist, who administered the gas, suddenly kicking the hinged wooden prop out from under the plywood, and I was immediately thrown into a horizontal position, strapped to the board. My reaction and response was not bad. I remember having a violent headache and felt disoriented, but I could hear screams from other cubicles near me. I chatted with some of the guys afterward, and their experiences were a lot worse. It was unreal. I think the whole thing lasted less than a half hour but seemed like an eternity. I don't believe the military would be allowed to do this today. Years later, the news of these secret tests was revealed by Art Eggleton, Canadian Defense Minister. In fact, in May of the year 2000, approximately two thousand Canadian armed forces personnel who had volunteered for the gas tests were honored by the unveiling of a plaque by Defense Minister Eggleton in Suffield, Alberta. As I think back and remember, it amazes to me how in spite of my headstrongness and my self-assurance and often my lack of acknowledging God in my life, He was there protecting me and even prodding me along the way. He was like a shepherd with wayward sheep. Today, and for a long time now, He's been my Shepherd King, and I am committed to go wherever He leads me!

Getting Out

After twelve weeks of intense, tough, and, I must say, valuable training, training that changed me from a boy to a man, I graduated from boot camp and headed to Camp Bordon to begin my course as an aircraftsman, second class as a safety equipment technician. I had no idea what that was! I arrived at Camp Borden, near Orillia, Ontario, on a cold winter day in early in February 1959. I was eager to begin this new course, but the course was not available, at least not yet. Meantime, I and the few guys who came with me washed military buses and cleaned latrines and stood around! It was boring, and I began to hate it. At night, everybody went to the bar but me. I didn't drink, and so I stayed behind in the barracks. I was lonely and felt discouraged. I began thinking about getting out, leaving the air force, but I had signed up for five years and so it seemed impossible. I wondered if God could help me with this. He could do the impossible. That's what my parents had taught me, and that's how they lived! But could He help me, and would He? I sure wasn't living my life for Him at that point!

My thoughts were continually consumed with a desire to leave Camp Borden, to leave the armed forces, to get back to my old life, to the shoe store and to my friends. I thought about it day and night. I even prayed about it occasionally. I finally spoke to my corporal, and he promised that he would have a word with the officers in my division. I figured it was worth a try, nothing ventured, nothing gained! Sometime later, I received an official order to appear before a board of officers. They grilled me on my reasons for wanting to leave the RCAF and did I realize that my commitment was for five years. I was honest with them and certainly humbled. In the end, I was released. I believe their reasoning was that it was peacetime, there was not a course available at Camp Borden for me at the time, and there was probably an abundance of other young men fresh from boot camp waiting to go on course. Maybe there were other reasons. But I am convinced that God had a plan for my life and that further time in the air force was not part of it. As I look back on the rest of my "journey," I can see this plainly.

Back to the Shoe Business

I returned to Etobicoke and was hired back at once by Lorne, my old manager at Pollocks Shoes, Cloverdale Mall, and went to live at Don's home. It was business as usual! Don's and my friendship never missed a step.

It was about that time that I met "Mall." Don and I had been constantly on the lookout for girls. We both needed a girlfriend. I don't remember exactly how we met, but I think Mall and her friend, Donna, came into Pollocks to buy shoes. Of course, I waited on them and was instantly attracted to Mall. We seemed to hit it off well, and as far as I was concerned, I was completely head over heels in love. This was the girl I would marry. After all, her whole family attended an Estonian evangelical church!

Mall was Estonian background and lived with her parents and sister a couple of miles northwest of Cloverdale Mall. I instantly nicknamed Mall Cloverdale Mall. Not sure she ever liked that! Her parents were very strict and not at all interested in my dating their daughter; besides, she was still in school. Our relationship lasted a year or two. I remember her calling me to tell me that she had met someone new; this broke my heart. I was desperately in love, and now it was over. I began praying at that time that God would bring someone into my life, a special girl who would love me and who would be His choice. I had no idea what He was about to do! It was amazing and still is!

Several months went by and then I was approached by Mr. Pollock asking me if I would consider managing a small store on Bayview Avenue. I jumped at the chance! I would be the youngest store manager in the chain. I had just turned twenty years old! This new challenge was strictly a commissioned position, 8 percent of sales. I hired and paid my own staff out of my eight percent, washed my own floors and windows, stocked my own shelves, shoveled my own snow, and everything else. I didn't have an assistant because I couldn't afford to pay one. So it was just me and the shoes and one part-time person who came in on Friday night and Saturday (when I could afford it). This was tough going! Some months were good, especially around Christmas; but January and February, the cupboard was bare, I mean bare! In those months, most weeks my weekend part-timer took home more than me. Then I got a phone call from Mr. Pollock telling me that he was closing the Bayview store and moving me to a new store in Oakville. I'm glad I'd persevered! It took me less time to drive to Oakville than it did to Bayview Avenue. I had a couple of part-time clerks but no assistant. The sales, however, were a little better; and my experience in managing people from the previous store and before that, with Lorne, proved most valuable. Managing people was often the most difficult part of the job. I believe God was teaching me how to be a "people person," one day at a time. I learned how to hire and fire, to encourage and challenge, and to say "thank you!"

During these early days, Don and I met Ron, a "kindred spirit," and Ron became a good friend. He lived just one street over and had a good job with Massey Ferguson. (I believe it was Massey Ferguson, but my memory is fuzzy about this.) We became three buddies, almost like the three musketeers. We hung out together, played pool together, and even bought brown suede jackets together. We were often seen heading for the mall, side by side, collars up, hair combed back like Elvis, swaggering as we walked. We were cool, man! There was one thing other than hanging out with us, which Ron liked to do. He loved his beer, and on weekends, after work on Friday, he would climb into his Beetle Volkswagen and drive a couple of hours to Honey Harbor where his parents had a cottage. He had many friends up there, and he would drink with them all weekend and return late Sunday night. Not sure how he managed to stay awake on the return trip late each Sunday.

A New Opportunity

Several months after moving to the Oakville store, I began to feel discontent. I was not moving ahead in my life, my future. I just wasn't satisfied as a shoe salesman or as shoe store manager. There had to be more out there, more challenge, more chance to move ahead, more money, and a better future. Don had a good job at a book-binding factory, making a lot more money than me.

The Tire Business

I noticed a building going up on Dundas Street West, close to where we lived. I found out that it would open soon, and it was to be a Dunlop Service Center. It had both a store and mechanical and installation bays. I applied as a retail sales clerk. After all, I was an experienced sales person and manager! However, I couldn't tell the difference between a car tire and a wheelbarrow tire! (Well, that's stretching it a little!) Dunlop needed a sales person and I got the job! Three weeks later, I was the retail manager. It was a retail/wholesale outlet, so not only did we sell and install tires and accessories to people who dropped in but also sold to service stations, tire dealers, and other distributors throughout a large region of southwestern Ontario. There were about ten or so employees at this location, including one guy on the road selling to distributors and one person driving a service truck, plus mechanics, installers, the general manager, and me. This was big business, and I was the retail manager! Now I was on my way. By the way, the pay was better and steady! I learned fast, and I enjoyed it!

One day, our wholesale man quit, and we hired a new one. He was a young fellow named Al. He needed a car. There was a Dunlop car available at our Ottawa location but he needed to fly there and drive it back. Al was deathly afraid of flying. I wasn't, so I offered to fly there and bring back the car. I'd never flown before in my life! Here was an adventure! The general manager agreed for me to go ahead, and so I did. It was the most exciting thing I'd done in my life. I'll never forget it. I think more importantly, my boss had the confidence in me and I so very much appreciated that. It was such an encouragement to me that someone, relatively new in my life, would trust me that way.

My Brother Evan

About that time, my brother Evan, my younger brother by three years, began attending Bible College in Toronto and needed a summer job. Dunlop was hiring students, and Evan applied and got the job. We decided it would be good to find an apartment together, and so we did, on the second floor of an old house! It was near High Park in West Toronto. We had a hilarious time together, rough-housing and having a ball! I remember one time we had made "Jell-O" in a plastic bowl and threw it back and forth between us to see who would miss it first. We each kept backing up, making the throw longer. I can't remember who won. I hadn't lived with any of my brothers since I was sixteen, and this reminded both of us so much of home.

As I look back, this was one of the most important decisions of my life. Evan was a strong believer and desired the Lord's best for his life. I, on the other hand, was marginal at best; but over the months, Evan's faith and his walk with the Lord had a profound influence on my life and my commitment. As I mentioned earlier, I had trusted Christ as a young boy of nine but never submitted my life fully to Him. Evan encouraged me to carefully consider where I was going and my testimony. Jesus Christ became my Lord and my King, and it was a result of my brother Evan's trust and his life. Such an example for me! I will forever be grateful to Evan! This was the beginning of a real change in me! Soon after, I began driving to Guelph every Sunday, and in time, the folks at Guelph Bible Chapel asked me to teach a Sunday school class of eleven- or twelve-year-old boys. These fellows grew on me. We hit it off well! And, as I prepared each lesson, I was growing in my understanding of the Bible and internalizing the truths that were there. I was growing like a new believer! My trust in Christ grew stronger and stronger. But there was much more to come!

As I grew in my faith, I became exceedingly more concerned about my buddies, Don and Ron. Neither were Christians, and this worried me greatly. I had shared to both about my faith and their need to trust Christ. I remember that there were special evangelistic meetings being held at the church in Guelph. I invited Ron to come with me on a Friday night instead of going north, and he said he would. We planned to meet on that Friday after work and drive to Guelph together. Ron called me the day before to tell me that he had changed his mind and that he would be heading north instead. That was the last opportunity I had to witness to my friend Ron.

Sunday School and My Bride-to-Be

In the fall of 1963, my Sunday school class along with the other grades was asked to prepare a presentation for our annual Christmas concert. So the boys and I put something together that included recitations and verses that they faithfully memorized for that evening. This was a big deal, especially for the boys and for me too! This was the first time in my life that I'd done something like this, except when I was a kid going to Sunday school myself. I loved memorizing and presenting to an audience!

I remember, in public school, I wrote a speech with the help of my dad on Alexander Graham Bell. I memorized it and still remember some of it! I came second in the whole class.

Anyway, that concert evening was another significant time in my life. My mother and dad were there along with many others including family, friends, and strangers. As I looked out over the audience, I spotted an amazingly beautiful girl. I had no idea who she was. After the concert and before the snacks, I asked my mother who this gorgeous girl was, because my mother seemed to know her. Mom told me her name was Beverley House; she was in nurses training for her registered nurse (RN) and was in Guelph for three months for her psychiatric training at the Homewood Health Centre. Since my mother knew her and I was busy with the boys, I asked her to see if I could drive Beverley back to residence after the evening was over. And so, my mother arranged my first date with my future wife! I tell people we met at a mental hospital but quickly confirm that I was not a patient! Beverley and I hit it off well, at least I thought so. I'm not sure Beverley was of the same mind. But she accepted my request for a second date. I believe we ended up at our family home where she had the "privilege" of meeting most of my eight brothers and two sisters. To say the least, she was overwhelmed, but she handled it well. I had to be constantly aware of my older brother; David was also on the lookout for a girlfriend. I was constantly on guard!

Well, it was love almost at first sight! Three dates later, I asked Bev to marry me, and she said "yes"! I believe she was taken completely by surprise, because she told me later that when she arrived at her residence, she said to herself, probably out loud, "What have I done?" Bev graduated the following spring as an RN from Toronto East General with a special award entitled "Award for Proficiency in Health Education." This was "The Joseph H. Harris Memorial Award." I was so very proud of her. At least one of us would have the brains in our family!

Excitement and Tragedy

Christmas 1963 was both an exciting time and a tragic time for me. On Boxing Day evening, I received a phone call from my old friend, Mall, to tell me that our friend Ron had been instantly killed in a car accident while heading home during a snowstorm, from Honey Harbor. I believe he had crashed head on into someone on Highway 400. Ron's mother and dad asked me to be a pallbearer for his funeral the following week. Don and I were shocked and heartbroken. To my knowledge, Ron never trusted the Lord.

Early the next year, I saved enough money to buy an engagement ring, a small diamond to be sure, a solitaire, but I knew that Bev would love it. I remember the evening at Bev's parent's home in Windsor, when I was about to slip the ring on her finger and, lo and behold, her mother walked into the room. But that didn't stop me! Just slowed me down a bit! I don't think that her mom knew our secret marriage plans, until then! We were now officially engaged, and we tentatively set our wedding date for the spring of 1965. That date got changed and so did a lot of other things!

Bev's Parents and Family

Joe and Helen House were Bev's dad and mom. They lived in Windsor, Ontario, several years where they started their family. They'd moved from Brantford years before and knew my parents, so when I was introduced by Bev, it wasn't a complete shock! They were amazing people and certainly loved their girls. Beverley was the middle sister, with Nancy being older and married to Bruce Cameron, and a younger sister Ruth, who later married Murray Martin. All three girls were very close growing up and remain so, to this day! Joe was working as an independent general insurance agent, and Helen was a stay-at-home mom. The House family was a close-knit family, so when I came on the scene, it was an interruption to be sure. But we did get along famously! I really came to love and appreciate each one in the family. They were so loving and patient and helpful especially during some of the difficulties we experienced. After Bev's graduation, she moved back home and nursed at one of the local hospitals until we were married in November 1964. Several years later, Joe became ill and spent about four years in hospital before he died on January 30, 1985. This was a difficult time for Helen and the girls, the daily trips to the hospital to feed and care for him. I will never forget Joe! He was one of my finest mentors, truly a man of God! Bev's mom struggled with several difficult health issues over the years. About 1993, Helen suddenly lost her eyesight and had to leave her apartment and spent the remaining five years in a senior's medical facility. Because Ruth and Bev lived hours away, Nancy had the bulk of the care for their mom. We will always be grateful to Nancy for her tireless commitment over those years. Their mom passed away on February 23, 1998. For me these many memories are valuable and stand out in my mind. It's just amazing to me how God puts families together and when hard times come His grace and His love are always sufficient!

Ottawa

I had no sooner arrived back in Toronto from that eventful "engagement" weekend when I received word from Dunlop that I was being transferred to the Ottawa branch. At first, I thought that our federal government was in trouble and needed my help. (I'm sure the Canadian government was in trouble, but they certainly didn't need help from me! In fact, they probably didn't know I existed!) But apparently Dunlop Ottawa needed me, and so I made plans to move there. Of course, the move was effective immediately! *Another amazing opportunity,* I thought! My future bride-to-be was shocked, to say the least. (I think my future mother-in-law needed oxygen!) But I was an adventurer, and Bev was just learning this! But she was also a trooper and still is to this day! God matched us well!

I got settled at a room and board place near Bank Street, close to the branch, and in the next few months; Bev made a train trip to Ottawa from Windsor, so we could go apartment hunting. In Ottawa, you needed to do that well in advance. It was frustrating and disappointing. There seemed to be nothing suitable in our price range. She went back home discouraged! Meantime, I had been at the Ottawa branch for about six months, did not like it much, and so requested a transfer back to the branch that I had come from. We prayed that God would grant this! He did! My old job was available, and I thankfully moved back! Bev was grateful too!

We moved the wedding date up from the spring of 1965 to November 14, 1964! We were deeply in love, but it was really me that convinced my bride with the earlier date. (I need to be honest about this!) She even gave up a scholarship she had won to further her nursing!

Growing in Love and in Christ

So we began our plans! At least Bev and her mother began the planning. The wedding ceremony and reception would be in Windsor, and I was just too far away. I loved Bev's dad, Joe! He was a great example for me, and I learned so much from him. I also immensely enjoyed her mother's cooking. It was always excellent. I hoped that Beverley could prepare meals like that! Helen, her mom, was a special lady, and she loved me! After all, I was about to become her son-in-law! Why shouldn't she? She was a wonderful cook and always had an amazing apple pie, freshly baked, just for me. (The others ate some too!) These memories are so valuable to me.

As I look back on my life, even at this point, I am truly amazed at how God Himself has cared for me and provided all that was needed along the way. It is indeed a mystery! No one could have even written the script. In many ways, at least at each moment, at each happening, at each incident, that seemed chaotic at the time, and without meaning, there was a thread intertwining through the days and years that brought meaning and purpose and direction in my life. Between the time of our engagement and the wedding day, I drove most weekends to Windsor from Toronto. Bev had moved back home after her graduation from Toronto East General and worked at Grace Hospital as an RN. Turner Road Gospel Chapel was her and her parent's home church, and we attended there and were married in that little church. During those months prior to the wedding, I was slowly growing in my faith and my commitment to Christ. Bev's family and the folks at Turner Road were a big part of that! We regularly attended the early Communion service, and I specifically remember one morning during worship time, the sun streaming through the windows while the congregation sang, each of us seated around the communion table. My heart was deeply challenged, not by just the words or the music but something much deeper. It was about the truth of the Savior's love and the enormous cost of my salvation, His life for mine! I was so overwhelmed, so thankful, that the tears began pouring down my cheeks. I tried to avoid anyone seeing, but I was so thrilled, so thankful in my spirit, so overjoyed that I almost could not contain it. I know for sure it was God's Spirit working and confirming in my heart that I was His and His alone and He loved me eternally and beyond comprehension! I'm reminded of the poem of the weaver written years ago, by an unknown author:

> My life is but a weaving
> between my Lord and me;
> I cannot choose the colors,
> He worketh steadily.
> Oft times He weaveth sorrow,
> And I, in foolish pride,
> Forget He sees the upper,
> And I the underside.
> Not 'til the loom is silent
> and the shuttles cease to fly,
> Shall God unroll the canvas
> and explain the reason why.
> The dark threads are as needful
> in the Weaver's skillful hand,
> As the threads of gold and silver
> in the pattern He has planned.
> He knows, He loves, He cares,
> nothing this truth can dim.
> He gives His very best to those
> who leave the choice with Him.
> (Author unknown)

Our Wedding

Well, the wedding day finally arrived! It was November 14, 1964. In spite of all the worrying about weather and rain, the day arrived sunny and glorious and warm! I wasn't worried in the least! I had asked God for this! I remember saying to Bev's mom not to worry about rain, just pray! I was admonished by her because I think I flippantly said to her, "Why pray when you can worry!" With all the concerns of preparations and planning, she didn't need my twisted humor. Anyway, she forgave me! I think!

All the details of the ceremony and reception are vague in my memory, but I do remember my beautiful bride coming down the aisle. She was gorgeous, white dress and all! Evan was best man and my brother David and Bev's sisters Nancy and Ruth were part of the wedding party. The reception was fun except for the part afterward when David and his friends Paul and Archie took me, physically, right in front of my new bride and rushed me into their car with the attempt to drive to Chatham (more than an hour way) and leave me on the street to find my own way back. I shouted and fought and complained bitterly until they had compassion, probably felt guilty and, after a few trips around the block, returned me to the reception hall and to my somewhat alarmed bride! Also, I remember our good friend, Ken, who was master of ceremonies, reading a letter to all of the guests and to Bev and I, of course. This was a letter that I'd written to Bev when I was fourteen. I had seen her and her sister earlier that summer at Guelph Bible Conference Grounds and was infatuated! I think I was the furthest thing from her mind at that point. Anyway, for some reason, she had kept my letter, found it a few months prior to November 14th, and showed to her mother who promptly gave it to Ken, master of ceremonies. I had no idea! Here's the letter:

August 29, 1954,
Guelph, Ont,
Box 777, O.A.C.

Dear Beverly,

From the back pages of an old scribbler, as I lie here on my bed, I am trying to compose a letter. First of all I will have to ask you to excuse my writing as I am in quite an awkward position, and secondly I hope you can translate some of these missing words.

Just think, only one more week before school starts. Won't that be ah . . . wonderful. My pen just ran out of ink and likely my pencil will break next.

David and Nancy had quite a time together this last week. For instance, on Saturday night after campfire, David said, "I suppose there isn't time for a walk," but there was, and I followed them for a while but soon lost tract of them. Don't tell Nancy that or she will tell my brother to hit me.

I sure wish I could see you again soon. Say you wouldn't happen to have a picture of yourself you could send me. I will try to hunt up one of me if you want it. Do you?

Do you know what? I have grown one-fourth inch since you saw me last. That makes me five feet and one and three-fourth inches. How tall are you?

David went to Detroit for a week to visit a friend, so he will probably come across to see Nancy.

Bev, please write me soon. I am dying to hear from you. Oh! Oh! Here comes Mom to shut off the light, so I must say goodbye.

Your good friend,
Richard Craig

This brought the house down! The other thing I remember about the wedding reception was that four of us sang the hymn "In Times Like These ." It was appropriate! Evan, Bill, Ken, and I had been singing in a quartet for the last year, and we decided that we would be part of the entertainment that day. It was hilarious and appropriate! Bev and I have many fond memories of that day!

We managed to escape, locate our car which was hidden in case my brothers found it, and we headed off on our honeymoon. Other than being chased by "friend" Dwaine, we made it safely to the Detroit border and crossed without incident and went on our way to Ann Arbor, Michigan. We were "beyond excited"! We had very little money, but thanks to Bev's mom (who'd saved all her "board money" for this event) and to her dad, for his credit card, we had an amazing trip down through Kentucky, Tennessee, North Carolina, The Smokies, and then up through Washington DC, Pennsylvania, and then New York State, back to Windsor and then to our new home in West Toronto.

Our First Home

Our first apartment was just a few miles from the Dunlop Service Center, where I worked. A couple of months before, Bev and I had found a small one-bedroom apartment that would be suitable for us newlyweds. It would be our first home. I was twenty-four, and she was twenty-three!

And so, we began life together! We were young and in love! Little did we know of what the future held for us! It was late November and Bev applied for a nursing position at a small hospital a few miles west of our home. There were no job openings at the hospital! I was shocked and upset when she returned to say that she'd offered to work on Christmas day. Our first Christmas together and she agreed to work? They offered to hire her because she was willing to work Christmas day! Nobody wanted to work on Christmas.

My friend, Don, was married close to that time as well. He seemed happy with his new bride and his new life although we didn't see him much.

My work at Dunlop was less challenging than before, and I kept thinking that I would like to find something that offered an opportunity to advance in business. I just needed a chance to show people what I could do. But I was not equipped in the accepted business sense nor with the right education. Who would hire me to work in an office? Bev and I talked about it often. She knew that I was dissatisfied and a bit discouraged, but she was always an amazing support for me. We prayed that God would provide something, somewhere.

In the meantime, we moved from our first place to a larger apartment with two bedrooms. It was a good price and gave us the extra room we needed.

Peterborough

I don't remember how this came about, but I heard about Fisher Gauge Works Limited in Peterborough, Ontario, a privately owned company that was in the zinc die casting business. The company was owned by David and Chester Fisher and started by their father many years before. Fisher produced and sold hundreds of configurations of small zinc castings used in telephones, automotive and aircraft instruments, business machines, and many other manufacturing applications. Fisher also developed, designed, and build die casting equipment which they sold all over the world. My dad's friend, George Reader, was secretary-treasurer of Fisher Gauge Works Limited! I decided that I would write him a letter asking if there were any employment opportunities in his firm!

To our surprise, he responded promptly, briefly outlining two job descriptions for positions that were open. One for which I was not qualified for at all, but the other, an entry-level position as an import/export customs clerk, seemed to offer some possibilities although I had no experience in that area at all! But it was worth a try! I phoned George Reader, and he and Helen graciously invited both Bev and I to come to Peterborough and stay with them. He promised to introduce me to those responsible for hiring at Fisher Gauge. Bev and I prayed that God would lead both them and us! I got the job!

As I look back, now, so many years later, I see clearly how God placed mentors in our lives, people who were men and women of faith to guide us and encourage us along the way. My brother, Evan, was one as were Ken and Thelma Shewell. So were George and Helen Reader! There were many more others along the way! I'll mention some of these as I continue my story. I strongly believe that each friend and mentor did not just happen, they were not just a coincidence in our lives, but they were strategically placed by God Himself. I'm sure you will see this as I continue!

Well, we gave notice at our apartment and our jobs and moved our few belongings from Toronto. We had found a small second-floor apartment in a house near Little Lake, in the heart of the city of Peterborough, Ontario. It was like little house on the prairie, but it was really little house on the lake. The folks who owned the place and lived on the ground floor were wonderful to us! Our young, married life had taken a new turn, and this amazing adventure together continued!

Bev applied and was hired by an ophthalmologist (an eye specialist) not long after we arrived. Prior to that, she'd worked as an RN for just a few weeks at the Peterborough General Hospital. Bev loved working for the eye specialist. It was really the perfect job for her!

We made many friends in Peterborough! We found a perfect church to attend and got involved in some of the opportunities there.

My job went well even though everything was new. I had taken a $25 weekly cut in pay to come to Fisher, but we really felt that the long-term opportunities outweighed the reduction in our personal revenue. God is faithful and the only way you can prove that is by looking back!

I worked with Fisher Gauge Works for almost one year. I learned so much about importing and exporting, of Canadian Customs documentations requirement, the rigger and the discipline required. I learned about international traffic and tariffs and transportation rates and the competitiveness of it all. It taught me something else about myself. It taught me that I had the mental capability to grasp these principles and to begin to understand how the commercial and industrial world works. But, oh, I had some much more to learn. When I moved on, I began to realize that I had barely scratched the surface. It was only the beginning!

New Opportunities

We received a call from Bev's dad. It was about midyear in 1965, and we'd been married less than a year! Bev's dad had a close friend, Joe, who was vice president and general manager (VP and GM) of Rockwell International in Tilbury, a small village east of Windsor, Ontario, where Bev's parents and Joe's family lived. The Rockwell division in Tilbury consisted of three separate companies under one roof and manufactured and assembled heavy truck components. Parts and materials for these were mainly imported from the United States and covered under the Automotive Trade Agreement tariff. Joe was looking for someone with experience in Canadian and US customs to be his traffic and customs manager for all three companies. Bev's dad had been talking to Joe about my work experience and my current job. I'm not sure if he mentioned how limited my experience was! Anyway, Joe wanted me to come to Tilbury for an interview. This was overwhelming to me. I had little education other than a small bit of hands-on experience. But I was eager to find out about it. I found out that Joe was a fine Christian and a brilliant VP and GM. He was well respected by his entire staff which included more than one hundred employees. Despite my marginal experience and lack of formal education, Joe offered me the position, if I agreed to attend the University of Windsor as an adult student to obtain a diploma in business administration. This would be done in the evenings and would take me six years to complete. I agreed!

Well, we packed up again for our move to Windsor! We had lived far from family since our marriage, but now we were going home, at least Bev was! We found an old fourplex to rent in the heart of Windsor. The rent was affordable, but the entrance to the place was dark and dreary. However, Bev, with her artistic ability, made our apartment bright and pleasant and warm! She immediately applied and was hired as a registered nurse at Grace Hospital, a Salvation Army Hospital in town. Her day shift was 7:00 a.m. to 3:00 p.m. but also was scheduled for afternoon and evening shifts occasionally. This certainly changed our lifestyle! I hated it when she worked weekends and evenings!

My new job was certainly a challenge! I was "green as grass!" For the first time in my life I was introduced to computer printouts, keypunching, and verifying. These terms are not recognized today, in this modern world, but back then it was "leading edge" technology! I did not do the keypunching, but part of my work was to analyze reams of printouts in relation to my work. Rockwell did not have a computer on site, so I often delivered stacks of prepared computer cards to our affiliate office in Windsor in the evening and returned to Tilbury the next day with printed reports and spreadsheets. I never saw it, but I was told that the massive computer in Windsor filled a whole room. We've come a long way!

My new boss at Rockwell was the manager of purchasing for the three Tilbury companies. His name was Carl, and he was very knowledgeable and helpful. We got along well. He taught me the ins and out of freight and freight forwarders and tariffs and introduced me to trucking company owners and personnel of key Canadian and US customs brokers on both sides of the border. It was indeed a "steep slope" of learning for me, a real challenge; but over the months, I learned it well and I enjoyed it immensely! I worked long hours including many Saturday mornings. I received constant support and encouragement from Joe! This meant a great deal to me!

In the meantime, I applied at the University of Windsor as an adult student, registered, and enrolled in their three-year business administration diploma program. I studied in the evenings and graduated six years later.

Rockwell International was a conglomerate of business enterprises spread out both in Canada and the United States. Rockwell, Tilbury, Ontario, was part of the automotive group with corporate offices in Troy, Michigan, located in the north part of the city of

Detroit. I traveled to Troy on two or three occasions during my time at Tilbury.

In the fall of 1966, Bev and I discovered that she was pregnant. We were excited beyond believe! We were going to be parents in June of 1967. It was going to be Canada's one hundredth birthday, and our first child was our personal "centennial project"! What a way to celebrate such an important national event.

For the first three or four months, Bev was quite sick, but she was a trooper, working every day regardless (and looking after me!). I'm afraid I wasn't much help! I remember coming home after work one evening to a dark apartment. When I opened the door, the savory aroma of roasted chicken caught my attention but no Bev! I found her in the back bedroom, in bed, under the covers. The smell of cooking chicken really turned her stomach! I ate the chicken!

Stephen

Finally, by the first of the new year (1967), Bev's sickness subsided; and together, we eagerly looked forward to June and the birth. Bev's younger sister, Ruth, was a student nurse at Grace Hospital where Bev worked, and Ruth was certainly intent on being part of the birth process. Bev and Ruth both knew the obstetrician, and so they figured they could pull some strings for Ruth to be in the delivery room. In those days, the fathers were not allowed anywhere near the "birth" room. Expectant fathers were relegated to a little waiting room down the hall, sort of "out of the way." After all, what did fathers have to do with anything?

Meantime, life went on! My job at Rockwell grew and became more involved as business increased. I wasn't sure what opportunities lay ahead, but I was confident that God would guide me; my faith was growing daily. I sometimes traveled back and forth from Windsor with Joe. He needed to leave his car for his wife occasionally, and so did I. These were good times together. He encouraged me in my walk of faith, but he was still the boss and I knew it; I respected him greatly! He was a tough manager. One time, I was in his office; and on his back credenza, I noticed a book entitled *Be Tough but Be Professional*. I've never forgotten that book and that title. That was exactly the way Joe was. There is no doubt in my mind and memory that Joe was one of my valued mentors and an amazing friend! What I saw in Joe was real!

On June 11, 1967, Bev informed me that we needed to head for the maternity ward. I drove her there along with her suitcase and my anxiety! Bev's parents and sisters were alerted, and my job was done! I was relegated to the little waiting room with the small TV. I had to stay quietly until the event occurred. Several hours later (it seemed that way at least), the door of the waiting room opened; and Ruth appeared holding this little bundle of humanity, just as he had been born, not even cleaned up. Ruth had been so excited to show me my son that she couldn't wait for anything. I remember I was thrilled and shocked! I'd never seen a newborn this new and in this condition before in my life. She took him away quickly, and after I had somewhat recovered my senses, I found my list of people to call. I remembered that I should call Bev first and congratulate her. Then I realized that she was the one who had the baby! Anyway, I recovered more of my senses and called our parents and family and then, anxiously, went down the hall to embrace my beautiful wife and my newborn son. Even the father, in these situations, goes through a lot of tumultuous and exuberant feelings and certainly anxiety! Bev was a mother, and I was a dad! We were so thankful to God for this incredible gift! But what a responsibility! Little did we know what the future held for us and for our newborn son. We had no idea how God would stretch us and support us and hold us up and show us His Majesty. We had so much to learn including our complete dependence on Him. Wow! What a lesson! And it was ongoing!

After about a week in hospital, Bev and Stephen arrived home to our little apartment. Then the fun began! Stephen did not nurse well. He cried constantly and kept us up night after night. We struggled those first few weeks wondering what to do. Our pediatrician told us that Stephen had colic which was related to an intestinal problem. Those were difficult weeks, especially at night, when Bev and I took turns walking the floor. I sang to him softly. It didn't seem to matter to him. At least, it kept me sane! We soon found out that his little legs at the hip joint were somewhat displaced in their sockets, so he was prescribed a special brace called a Denis Browne bar to keep his hips and legs straight. This was treatment for what they diagnosed as hip dysplasia. It was essentially a bar attached to the sole of a pair of little boots. This apparatus was to be worn at night while he slept. I was so thankful that I was married to an RN with a heart of gold. I never would have made it on my own!

Advancement

At about this time, I was called into the VP and GM's office to meet with Joe. He informed me that he was pleased with my progress as his traffic and customs manager working with and for Carl. He also informed me that Carl had been offered and accepted an opportunity to work at the corporate offices in Troy, Michigan, as international procurement officer. Carl would be leaving shortly, and Joe asked if I would consider taking on the role of purchasing manager for Rockwell, Tilbury. He said that he felt I could fill this role and Carl would train me in his remaining time at Tilbury. I was absolutely flabbergasted!

I had no experience in buying except, maybe, buying my own socks! But Joe felt I could do this. He said that the key thing in his decision was that he knew he could trust me. Here's a guy with limited education that was being offered a middle-management position in a major company, to serve under one of the finest and sharpest VPs that I had ever met. I said "yes" to Joe! The next three or four years were the most challenging and most rewarding years in my business life, so far!

Many people wonder if God really exists and if He really cares for us, personally and individually. I'm absolutely convinced that He does. I firmly believe that it has to do with knowing Him and trusting Him. Although my faith in Him is weak at many times, I believe that God is the God of Heaven, that He is the Sovereign God, and that He Himself was and is in charge of my life and so does Bev. It is because we have placed our trust totally in Him alone. In the Bible, in New Testament, in the book of Hebrews 11 (I call it the faith chapter), this is recorded in verse 6:

> And it is impossible to please God without faith. Anyone who wants to come to him must believe that God exists and that he rewards those who sincerely seek him. (Hebrews 11:6, NLT)

As my story continues, over the next forty plus years, you will see that this is true!

It was 1967! What a year! Canada's Centennial Year! The job and the new responsibilities were going well! I was very anxious to please but also wanted people to know who I was and what I stood for. God gave me the confidence, but I sure needed assurance from others. My greatest ally was Bev; she was behind me all the way. I think the saying goes: "Behind every great man is a great woman!" I believe that's especially true of the husband in Proverbs 31.

Verses 10–12 say this:

> Who can find a virtuous and capable wife?
> She is more precious than rubies.
> Her husband can trust her,
> and she will greatly enrich his life.
> She brings him good, not harm,
> all the days of her life.

Challenges

When Stephen was just a few months old, we detected that Stephen did not seem to respond to sound. For a while we just thought it was our imagination, but as we continued to watch, we grew concerned. Our pediatrician assured Bev when she questioned him that his hearing was okay and not to worry. Bev persisted with the pediatrician, and finally, after a few months, we were put in touch with an audiology specialist in Detroit, Michigan. We proceeded, with great concern, to take Stephen for testing. Before Stephen was a year old, it was concluded by the audiologist that he was profoundly deaf. Even though, in a way, we had sensed this diagnosis for some time, it hit us hard. *What does profound deafness mean? Could it be treated? What was the prognosis? What do we do now?* All these questions captivated our thoughts. *How do we handle this one? What do we do for our son? Why, God?* I remember praying, "Lord, how do I communicate with my son and he with me. Lord, how will I ever tell him about you?" So many questions and so few answers. Fortunately, we had an amazing family, who were and are incredibly supportive. We were just a young couple with a deaf son.

I am a "fix it" person at heart. If it's broken, I'll fix it. It's in my nature. But I couldn't fix Stephen! I found out that nobody could. "Lord, this is a mountain for us and for our beloved son!"

We received lots of advice from the audiologist in Detroit, about things to do to help with communication. For instance, hold Stephen on our knee and show him simple pictures of things like a ball or a truck or a dog and say the word out loud by putting his little hand on our cheek and by looking into his eyes. This way he could see our mouth form the words and feel the sound of our voice. Bev spent hours and hours doing this. She had hundreds of pictures. The specialist arranged for a hearing aid and we had molds made for each of his ears. We bought expensive "vocalizers"(children's hearing aids), an apparatus that we hung first on his back and encouraged him to listen. When that didn't work, we put the aid on his chest in a harness that we called a bra. The hearing aid had a cord leading to the earmold in his ear. He received his first hearing aid for his first birthday! The second one came a few months later. After a year or so, we realized that these aids, although powerful, were not effective at all. Stephen received no sound at all! He could only feel vibrations and what he heard through his eyes. At about the same time, we noticed that there seemed to be a weakness in his eyes with one eye turning in. An Ophthalmologist instructed us to patch the "good eye"! This would allow the weaker eye to strengthen. We went through this for a year, first patching one eye with an adhesive patch; and when the other seemed to turn in, we switched to patching it. On Stephen's second birthday, he had eye surgery to correct the problem. Bev was allowed to go in with him wearing her nurse's uniform and was allowed to stay extended hours but not overnight. I remember his surgery, the anxious waiting and then leaving him overnight at the hospital. Of course, he was sedated, and we needed to sleep.

As we entered his ward early the next morning, we heard dry sobs from his small hospital crib. Stephen was standing, holding on to the rail, his eyes bandaged and no hearing aid. Bev rushed to pick him up and embrace him. He knew it was his mom immediately, and he burst out crying and clung to her for dear life. It is a memory that will never go away!

David and Nancy

In the fall of 1967, an amazing thing happened that made a tremendous impact on my life. I remember that I was glancing through *The Windsor Star* newspaper one evening after dinner and a small article caught my eye. The headline read: "Canadian Missionary Faces an African Firing Squad." The first line began, "Reverent David Trevor Craig faces firing squad in Nigeria"! I suddenly realized that they were writing about my brother! This was such a shock to me. I had known Dave and his wife, Nancy, were in Nigeria serving with the Presbyterian Mission. I learned later that he'd recently been appointed chaplain of the Hope Waddell Training Institution in the port city of Calabar. He also served as pastor to six churches in that city and nine in the bush. Together, Dave and Nancy served and loved the Nigerian people. Calabar is in the eastern region of Nigeria, about 130 miles from the Cameroon Republic. Apparently during the previous year, Lt. Col. Odwumegwo Ojukwu declared the region the independent Republic of Biafra; and ever since, there had been fierce fighting between the Biafrans and the Nigerian federal forces. As the fighting grew more intense, foreign business people and others were encouraged to leave the country. Dave insisted that Nancy leave as well, but David felt it was God's will that he should stay. As the war became more intense and moved closer to Hope Waddell, supplies dwindled and Dave and a friend went in search of food. Soon after, they were captured by Nigerian troops. The leaders stated that Dave was a Chinese mercenary working with the Biafrans. Dave told them he was a missionary, not a mercenary, but they would not listen. They had heard there were mercenaries fighting with the Biafrans. (Mercenaries are professional and dangerous soldiers and fighters who hire themselves out to whoever pays the most.) Some of the black soldiers fear them, believing they have "Juju" or special magic power.

They took Dave and his friend to the entrance to a courtyard of a large cement factory. The whitewashed gate was smeared with blood. So were some of the outside walls of the factory. Groups of soldiers in sweat-soaked battle dress pressed closer wanting a close look at this one deadly specimen, this live mercenary. The two prisoners were commanded to sit back to back on the ground. The NCO shouted to the soldiers, "Take your positions," and the soldiers formed a wide circle around them.

Someone shouted, "If you are not a mercenary, why did you stay when you were told to get out?"

Dave responded, "Because God asked me to stay with His people in their trouble."

"You'll stay, all right!" another voice called out. The soldiers began cocking their weapons, and Dave told me later that he heard safety catches clicking off.

"May God forgive you!" Dave called out and bowed his head to pray.

"Lift up your head! Open your eyes!" they yelled. Dave said later the rifles were pointing at them. They were taking aim. He could see the hatred and loathing on the men's faces.

Suddenly, a voice yelled, "Stop!" It was the batman of the commanding officer. "The colonel wants to see him." The soldiers were not pleased, but they obeyed the order. God had again done an amazing thing! There is much more to this story, perhaps for another time. My conversations with Dave and Nancy and the stories of Africa, the people, and their love for them deeply affected me and my own walk with God. What an example for me!

(*Note:* Most of Dave's story is from details I remember in my many talks with Dave and Nancy, and some are from *The Windsor Star* Weekend Magazine publication dated January 27, 1968.)

Advancement

My new position at Rockwell International, Tilbury, continued to progress under the excellent leadership of Joe. He was demanding and tough but always fair, not just to me but to all his employees. Joe was highly respected throughout the organization and certainly by me! I felt valued! My confidence grew as I learned the job. I developed techniques for buying and negotiating. I met with manufacturers and service providers. I was also learning a great deal through my studies in finance, economics, and personnel management at the University of Windsor. It was grueling at times, keeping all "the balls in the air," between work, my growing family with special needs, my university studies, and my church activities. My wife, Beverley, was such a wonderful support to me; and she had so much on her plate, including nursing part-time at the hospital, looking after Stephen with his many medical appointments and special needs that he had, plus the up-keep of our home and meals. I will be forever grateful to her, for her partnership and her endless love. Her mother and dad were so very helpful and supportive, in countless ways. They often took Stephen and cared for him, while Bev was working and to give us a break.

Home Ownership

Bev's dad worked as a general insurance agent and sold insurance to both individuals and small businesses. One of the businesses was a small contractor who built small homes in the area. We were introduced to him and with Bev's dad's help arranged for him to build us a little split-level home at the edge of a golf course. We had found the property, and the contactor agreed to buy the land and build a house for us. Our very first house and it was brand new. The contractor agreed to carry a second mortgage for us for three years, and along with a small loan from Bev's mom and dad, we were able to swing it! To us, it was amazing! Besides, we were expecting our second child, so we needed the extra space. This, surely, was another gift from God.

Oakwood

My responsibilities at our small church included, with others, arranging for speakers plus some planning for special music. Oakwood Bible Chapel in Windsor, Ontario, was where we worshipped. Oakwood is an independent Bible Chapel without a formal pastor but, rather, overseen by elders. There are many of these "assemblies" throughout North America with able Bible teachers. Each Sunday throughout the year, we had either special guest speakers come for other communities as preachers for the day or, often, qualified men from our own church.

Bev and I had met Doug, an Evangelist from the Peterborough area when we lived there during our first year of marriage. We had helped counsel at Graphite Bible Camp in the Kawartha Lakes area, north of Bancroft, a kid's Bible camp that Doug had founded some years before. Doug was the hands-on camp director!

Our committee at Oakwood Chapel invited Doug to come as guest speaker, for a series of Evangelistic meetings. Doug stayed with Bev, Stephen, and me. Doug was one of my mentors. I will never forget him, especially his counselling that week when he stayed with us. He was very industrious and always wanted to "pay his way." I remember his kneeling on our living room floor, upholstering our worn couch. Stephen was perhaps a year or so, and Doug could see his struggles and ours. As I was watching Doug work, he suddenly looked up at me and said, out of the blue, "Dick, do you ever ask God to increase your love for your wife?"

I was a bit taken back, but I responded saying, "I don't think I've ever thought about that, Doug!"

Then he said, "You need to begin doing that and you need to start today!"

For some time, I thought that this counsel was kind of strange, but I began to pray as he had said. As I look back over almost fifty years, I realize how valuable and wise his instruction had been for me. As I prayed this simple request to God, I began to realize that my prayer should be, "Lord, please increase my love for you!" As I prayed this request to God, Bev's and my relationship began to blossom and grow! As I prayed, the Lord began to thrill me, more and more, with His presence and grace in my life. This has developed and grown in my life over these many years. I will be forever grateful to Doug Robinson, my mentor and friend!

Carolyn

March 20th of 1971 was a day to remember! Almost everyone thought Bev was going to have another boy. This time I was allowed in the delivery room. Times had changed! Fathers were now allowed to witness their babies being born!

As our baby's head and shoulders appeared, we were sure it was another boy, at least I was! But it wasn't a boy! Our beautiful daughter, Carolyn Ruth, came into the world! We were so thrilled! God had given us one of everything! First a son and now a daughter. We had the perfect family. She was a beautiful baby!

As we have watched her grow and mature over the years, Bev and I are so thankful for her. Now, as we observe Carolyn as a mom of two of her own amazing daughters, we truly see God's hand in her life and in ours, and we love her even more!

Communication

Communication with Stephen continued to be difficult. Stephen made noises, guttural sounds, but had no speech or words. Touch, gestures, facial expression, and hugs were our only means of interaction with him. We were so very concerned about the future. How would he ever get along in this world? His hearing aids did not seem to help him at all. I remember crying out to God! "Lord, how will we ever be able to tell him about you? We can't even communicate with him!" This is just the beginning of an amazing story, at least amazing to us, of God's faithful care.

Before he was four years old, we enrolled Stephen at Victoria School in Windsor, a special school for hard of hearing and deaf children. Early each morning, Bev would help him into a special taxi with his backpack, lunch, and snack for his ride to school. The taxi driver would return him home, midafternoon. This was a very difficult time for Stephen and for us. At first, we thought this would help him but came to realize that this school was not the answer. In fact, much later, we realized that it was more damaging than good!

Meantime, our new little baby girl had problems of her own. She was often congested and had trouble breathing. At one point, Carolyn stopped breathing, and Bev had to run to the neighbors for help. They rushed them to the doctor. Carolyn's health challenges continued until her pediatrician discovered that she was struggling with several different allergies. She certainly has had a difficult time over these years.

My work was more than a half hour drive from home, so I was of no help. I would never have been able to cope if it wasn't for my amazing wife! I will always be thankful and grateful for Bev, for her wisdom and her unwavering faith in God, for her gentleness, and for her courage! One of my favorite Bible verses says it all:

> A wife of noble character who can find?
> > She is worth far more than rubies.
> (Proverbs 31:10)

It was 1972 and we knew that we had to investigate what to do about Stephen's schooling. There seemed to be only two options. One was to send him to a residential school for the deaf in either Milton, Ontario, or Belleville. The other option was to move to either of these cities where he could live at home and attend school as a day student. The first option meant us putting our six-year-old son on a yellow school bus on Sunday afternoon for a four-hour ride to school residence and then not seeing him again for one or two weeks. We knew that this was not for us or for Stephen.

My work at Rockwell International was going well, and the business opportunities seemed promising, but our growing family was priority number one. We prayed regularly and often, asking God what to do. We sure had no idea! Then we learned that the Ontario provincial government was building a new residential school for the deaf in London, Ontario. It would be called Robarts School for The Hearing Handicapped and would be opening in January of 1974. This seemed to be a better answer for us, but still, Stephen would have to live in residence away from his family. Again, Bev and I cried out to God about this! *What should we do?* There is a scripture that stands out in my mind as I recall and write this. Perhaps it's often overused, and often misapplied, but I believe it is appropriate here. The Bible is our guide book, and it's full of promises for us and for those who trust in Him. In my mind and in my heart, there is no question that these verses apply in our lives because we have proven them to be true:

> For I know the plans I have for you," declares the LORD,
> > "plans to prosper you and not to harm you,
> plans to give you hope and a future."

MY LIFE DOES IT REALLY MATTER?

Then you will call on me and come and pray to me,
    and I will listen to you.
    You will seek me and find me
    when you seek me with all your heart.
(Jeremiah 29:11–13, NIV)

Confidence

Even though I had advanced in business, I struggled with confidence, really an inferiority complex. I had no difficulty speaking one-on-one with my colleagues and peers or even meeting with suppliers, but I could not speak in front of an audience. My self-esteem was as low as it could be. Even in seminars, I was fearful of being centered out, of being asked to respond to a question, and I was devastated when ever asked to take the lead in a discussion group. In fact, I was terrified.

A few months before their wedding, Bev's sister, Ruth, and fiancé, Murray, came to me asking that I be master of ceremonies for their wedding. I refused, I said I just can't speak in front of people, but they just wouldn't take no for an answer. I was terrified! I just couldn't do this, but I didn't have an "out." I spent hours and hours looking up jokes and memorizing lines, especially the "punch lines"! Finally, the day came and the whole thing went well, at least everyone said so, and they laughed at my stories and jokes. I was amazed and so thankful! Probably thankful because it was over, and I didn't drop the wine glass when I was toasting!

This was one of the best things that ever happened to me. Over these last forty-some years, I have spoken at conferences and churches, funerals, and weddings and have preached to congregations in several places in and out of Ontario. I will always be thankful to Ruth and Murray for encouraging me and "pushing me" with gentleness and firmness!

Moving Again

Bev and I did seek counsel from her mom and dad and mine and others. It became clear that Stephen should attend Robarts School in London and that our family should move to that city. That way, Stephen could live with his family and not in a residence. Of course, this meant major changes in all our lives. We had to find a job, pull up stakes, find a house, and all of that! I put together a resume and began the job search. At least I had my university business diploma this time and seven years of successful business experience with a major automotive manufacturing company.

In only a few weeks, I was offered a position as purchasing manager with a London-based crane manufacturer named General Crane Industries. The pay was substantially less, but it would meet our needs, and the opportunities for growth and advancement seemed possible. We found a house, sold our Windsor one, and moved in time for Stephen to begin at Robarts School. Our new life in London had begun! It was like starting over! It was the end of January 1974. Stephen was six and a half years old, and Carolyn was about to turn three! She was becoming such a great help to her mom!

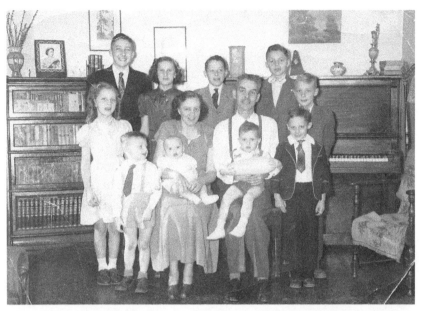

The Craig Family *minus* Ian – (*Not Born Yet*)

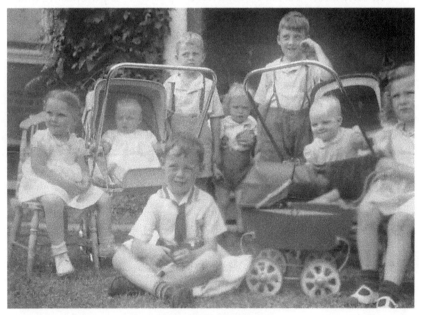

Dick – 'In Charge!'

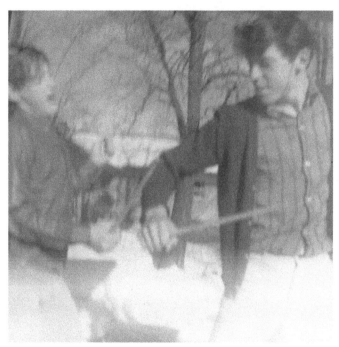

Youngest brothers Ian (*On Left*) & Mark 'A Brotherly Duel'

Growing Up

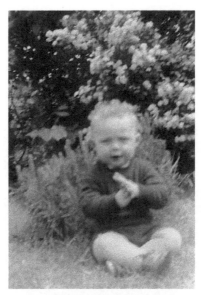

Dick (Richard)
at 1 1/2 years old

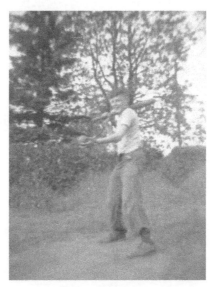

The Sportsman

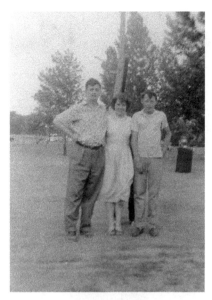

Dick (Richard)
with Friends

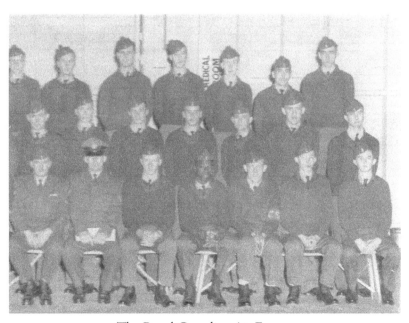

The Royal Canadian Air Force -
Dick – First Row, second from Rig

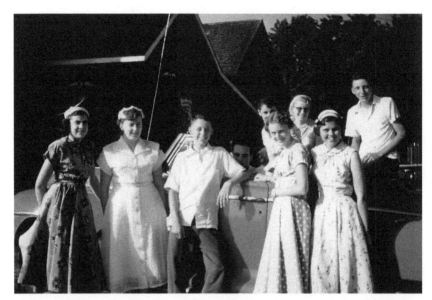

Dick (*middle*) & Friends Oldest Brother David – Far Right

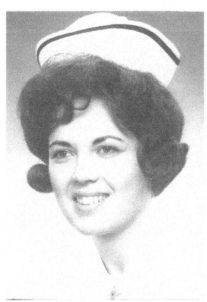 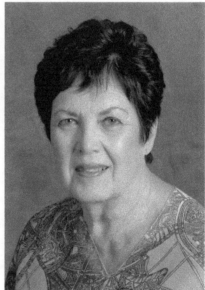

Beverly – Then & Now

MY LIFE DOES IT REALLY MATTER?

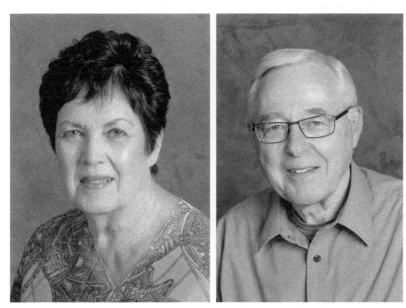

Me and My Bride

DICK CRAIG

Our Daughters, Son & Sons-in-Law

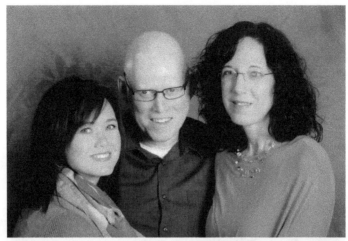

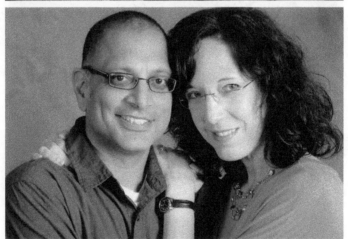

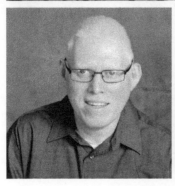
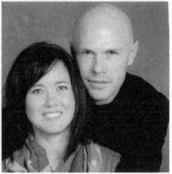

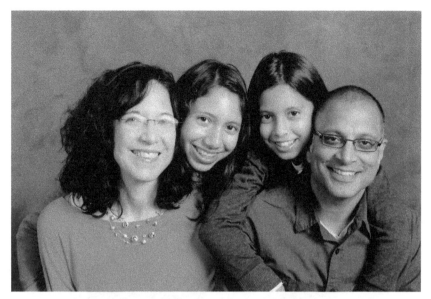
Daughter Carolyn & Indy Jaswal with children Emma & Maya

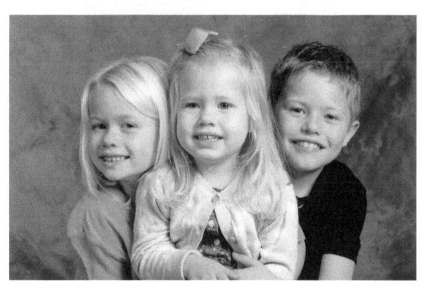
Enns Children Georgia, Charli & Jaxson

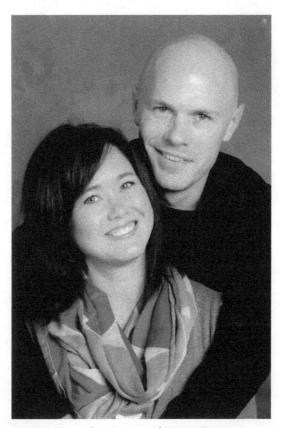

Daugther Janis with Sean Enns

Mark

My mother and dad also moved that year from Guelph to Sundridge, Ontario, a small town south of North Bay. Dad had taken retirement at age sixty-six from his work at the college in Guelph. Just a few months later, my brother, Jim, phoned me from his home in South River with the tragic news that our second youngest brother, Mark, had choked to death in his sleep. Mark was twenty years old and had recently begun an autobody mechanic apprenticeship in Carleton Place, a small town near Ottawa, Ontario. The news was devastating to us all, especially to our dad and mom. This was the first break in our family. None of us had experienced tragedy like this before. We all felt lost without Mark. Our hearts were broken, especially Mom and Dad's. There were thirteen of us including our parents. Now there were twelve!

General Crane Industries

General Crane Industries was a fascinating new company and challenge for me. This company was privately owned, and its principals designed, engineered, and built huge hydraulic mobile tower cranes that folded into a specially built forty-eight-foot trailer bed (also specially designed), pulled by a large diesel tractor. The crane tower included three different sized lattice sections, the smaller two tower sections inserted inside the larger ones and held together by a giant cylinder. When raised from the trailer bed vertically and fully extended, the tower's height stood more than 120 feet in the air, a huge platform and 80-foot boom mounted on its top. In addition, there were two lattice boom extensions, one forty feet and one twenty feet, attached on the side of the trailer. These were available at the job site, should extra reach be required. I'm told, when all assembled and ready, the crane was 332 feet tall. A massive thing!

My job was to buy special steel and hydraulic components for these things! I knew nothing about cranes and hydraulics and engineering and drawings. *Wow, Lord, what have I got myself into?* Maybe a better prayer was, "Lord, how am I ever going to do this?" I worked directly for the president and owner of the company. He was patient and an excellent teacher. I traveled with him to meet with many suppliers and designers. He taught me how to know and read and understand engineering specifications and how to interpret complex drawings. I learned quickly under his watchful eye. I certainly did appreciate him, his knowledge and his expertise. He allowed me to make mistakes, and I made many of them! But gradually I learned the business. The market for these cranes was both United States and Europe. Each unit sold for more than $250,000. After a few years, the owners sold the entire company to Grove Crane Manufacturing (now known as Manitowoc), a worldwide crane designer and builder with head offices located in Shady Grove PA. I got along well with the new president who also took me under his wing. He seemed to have confidence in me from the beginning, and my self-confidence was growing as well. But always in the back of my mind was the thought that the people I worked with and the people I worked for were so much better educated than I was. *Smarter too,* I thought! This often bothered me. I often felt inadequate. I was working in a world surrounded by competent, highly educated people with university degrees, and I felt inferior.

But again, I believe that God was with me each step of the way and that He would never ever let me down! I know this today, for sure! It's not imagination or coincidence or luck. It's just knowing that He is always there with me and for me. And so, I trust in Him. He is my all in all!

I often think of acquaintances and friends and family who don't yet know Him, as I do. I cry out to God in my spirit for them that they would simply trust Him! I know it's worth it all!

Our beautiful little girl, Carolyn, started school. Our house backed unto the school grounds, so it was easy for Bev to walk with her to kindergarten each day. Stephen, on the other hand, was picked up each morning by cab and transported right across London to the northeast side, to Robarts School. Carolyn was brilliant at school, right from the beginning. Stephen learned finger spelling quickly and adjusting to a new school with a different philosophy of learning. It was so different from Victoria School in Windsor. There were many challenges for him. Bev and I took a "finger spelling" course and began to learn how to speak with our son using our hands. With "finger spelling," the person speaking spells out each letter of each word using their fingers. It takes a long time to say something, but it's effective. We practiced for months, forming the twenty-six alphabet letters with our hands and memorizing the shape of each letter. At Robarts School, Stephen was not allowed to learn or use ASL (American Sign Language) during his time there. In his fourth grade, Signing Exact English was introduced where the exact structure of a sentence is signed. This means signing or finger spelling every word in a proper sentence including connecting words like "but" or "and" or "the" and others. ASL is short for American Sign Language and is commonly used for communication by the deaf in North America. ASL includes a hand sign for every conceivable word, and if a sign doesn't exist, the deaf will make one up. Early on, Stephen made a special sign for his name, using the "S" symbol with his right hand on his forehead and then on his chin. Of course, most of the deaf picked this up in an instant!

Deaf people using ASL most often leave these connecting words out in their communication with each other. They don't find them necessary.

Later, we found that communication was much faster using signs! Stephen did not learn or use ASL with expertise until after he left secondary school and began college.

We gradually learned that total communication is much more than finger spelling and signs. It also includes facial expressions, body language, and using the other senses. Even vibrations are a part of it. When we want Stephen's attention at home, we'll often stomp on the floor. He feels the vibration, and he turns to us. Later, Bev and I began learning sign language as well. Carolyn was a "wiz" at finger spelling, and even at a young age, she was so helpful with Stephen. She is one of God's specials gifts to Bev and me!

As our children developed and grew in our new home in London, Ontario, I continued to progress in my work at General Crane Industries. There were many challenges along the way. At the same time, I kept my eye open for fresh opportunities.

We certainly had a busy household during those "London" days! Carolyn and her friend, Brenda, who just lived up the street, were involved in gymnastics. They loved practicing and developing their skills at a local gym and in the backyard. Bev was busy with family, running them here and there, helping at school, involving in Bible studies, as well as working with Stephen on developing his communication skills. She also served in the church nursery and junior church. I met with leaders of Boy's Christian Service Brigade at Wortley Baptist, where we attended as a family. I wanted Stephen, despite his deafness, to be a part of this boy's group. The leaders asked me to participate and be the communication link for my son. They were a fine bunch of guys, and even though Stephen had no speech and was profoundly deaf, he was accepted and included as one of them. It didn't take long before many of the boys not only learned but became proficient at finger spelling, and they were the communicators. Most of the time, they didn't even need me as they went through their lessons and tests. Stephen is still friends with one or two of these guys even to this day. At Wortley Baptist, I joined a men's choir; and over a few years, we were invited to sing in several churches throughout the area. I remember we joined with three other groups of men and sang at Hamilton Place. There were about one hundred of us in all, singing great hymns of the faith, all a Capello. It was an amazing musical evening, just these talented men and two pianists called the Bowker Brothers, each playing a grand piano. It was an amazing night. The men could blend and harmonize and fill that huge hall with music and praise. It was an evening to remember.

Bev and I served in the church library and had other responsibilities over the years. Carolyn and Stephen attended Sunday school at Wortley. Bev and I took turns siting in with Stephen to translate the lesson for him.

I also attended evenings at Fanshawe College, London, where I took several business-related courses including marketing and inventory and production planning. I was successful in completing and passing each of them.

London is a university town with a mix of professional and manufacturing businesses. General Motors and 3M were the major "anchor" companies with Ford Motor Company in nearby St. Thomas. Also, London was home to several financial headquarters and legal establishments. In addition, the highly acclaimed University of Western Ontario (UWO) and University Hospital, a major teaching hospital, are in London as well.

At General Crane, under new ownership and management, my responsibilities increased. As well as my purchasing duties, I was asked by the new president to assume the role of office manager, overseeing finance as well as buying. The office staff was small, but we worked well together. At Christmas, I received a generous bonus from the president. The following year, business seemed to slow down, and I wondered just what lay ahead.

Excello

Several months into the new year, an opportunity came up, again in the manufacturing sector, with a company that designed and built progressive machining and assembly lines, mainly for the automotive industry. This was a much larger company than General Crane Industries, and to me it seemed to offer more opportunity for advancement. The company's name was Excello Corporation, also located in London, Ontario. Excello had several sister companies in Windsor, Ontario, and in the United States. The London location had advertised for a general purchasing manager, so I applied. I was interviewed by the VP and GM and was offered the position! I submitted my three-week notice to the president of General Crane, and he seemed greatly concerned. A week or so later, he called me into his office to say that he was disappointed that I was leaving but he understood my decision. He stated that he was very pleased with my work and gave me a $500 bonus. I was absolutely overwhelmed that he would do this. I have never ever forgotten this, and I will always be grateful to him!

Well, this new beginning and the events that followed that year and the next were mind-boggling, at least to me. My job at Excello was to oversee eleven purchasing staff in both general and subcontract buying. There were two supervisors, one in each department, plus buying clerks and secretaries. This was indeed a challenge. Both supervisors were my senior and had been with Excello for a long time. I was just a young guy from "outside" who probably didn't know much! I realized early that I had to work alongside them and gain their confidence and make them see that they were highly valued. This took a great deal of time and effort. It was very troubling at times and difficult, but over the course of several months, things began to come together. I constantly prayed for God's wisdom and His strength. How I needed this and the encouragement of my dear wife!

Not only did I have a staff to win over, but I had a business to learn. Part of my job was to work with a team of engineers, mechanical design people, hydraulic and pneumatics specialists, and electrical experts. There were about twenty-five of them! And I knew nothing about special machinery. These guys and girls were great to me! They virtually taught me what a "progressive machinery line" was and how it worked. These complicated machines were sold to customers as a concept from an engineering drawing. Our customers were companies like Ford Motor and General Motors and Caterpillar Inc. and Chrysler Corporation and others. Excello's team of specialists virtually designed, built, and tested the equipment on the factory floor, then shipped it to the customer's plant, where our people assembled it completely and proved it again on the customer's factory floor. Lead time was anywhere from eighteen months to three years. This equipment was valued at anywhere from $2 to $4 million. It was big business, and I was in the "middle of it"! My learning curve was steep! As I look back now, I'm astonished that a shoe salesman, an ex-military jock, a guy with one-year high school, could go this far. Or even more surprising is how was it possible that so many different people had the confidence and trust in me, to allow me to come this far. To me, it's a miracle! And you know something? It is! I have no place and no one to acknowledge this except to God, Himself. He, indeed, is my Majesty! He has shown me His incredible grace and blessed me with His wisdom! I will forever praise Him!

But it's not over yet! There's more!

Janis

A year or so after my joining Excello, several things happened. It was 1976. I was thirty-six years old. In the fall of that year, Bev and I received the news from her doctor that Bev was pregnant and that we would have an addition to our family the following May. This was a pleasant surprise, having a third child in our "old age"! On May 5, Janis Ann came into the world, a baby sister for Carolyn and Stephen. There was excitement in our house! A second beautiful daughter! Another precious gift from God! Janis was the only one of our children born on a working day. There was concern of distress at her birth, so our pediatrician was called in and at one point five medical people surrounded Bev's bed. But Janis was born without any problem, and I was able to be in the room! We are so thankful for her and thrilled as she raises her handsome son and two beautiful daughters.

In the meantime, at Excello things began to change for me. The annual sales of our division were just over $12 million, and the order board was increasing annually.

I was asked by the VP and GM, my boss, to take on the role of materials control manager. This was a new position for Excello Corporation. I was being asked to become part of the senior management team of the London division. As materials control manager, I would be responsible for overseeing and managing not only purchasing but also production planning, inventory control, traffic, customs, and factory stores. This meant the responsibility of seventy employees including five supervisors. Now, here was a challenge! I accepted the role! It was exciting and political to be sure. I was not a politician in the least and didn't even know how to be one! This was the most frustrating part of the management role for me. But, somehow, I survived!

Excello, London, had more than three hundred employees, and we were "splitting at the seams" in terms of space. To the east side of the factory, there was a large piece of Excello land available for expansion, and we needed more assembly floor. Corporate decided to expand. The management team put together a plan, detail drawings were completed by an engineering firm, and we were ready to search out three potential building contractors for quoting on this project. The budget was about $2.2 million. When the decisions were made to proceed, the VP and GM called me into his office. As you know, my plate was already full with my new position and responsibilities and my boss knew that! As I sat at his boardroom table, he looked into my eyes and said, "Dick, I want you to oversee this building project for me, including recommending which contractor we should use, buying two overhead cranes, working with the lead construction supervisor on a daily basis, and making sure that every drawing detail is correctly carried out. You will report to me daily on the progress, and you will not exceed the $2.2 million budget!"

To say the least, I was flabbergasted! I knew nothing about construction, about building a building. Why would he choose me to be the leader on this project? Why not our chief engineer or the head of our design department? Why me? I think it was because he knew that I would do my best and that he trusted me. I tried to be reliable in the past. Also, I had excellent and trustworthy and experienced supervisors in each department that I was responsible for in the material control function.

I accepted this new challenge! There is nothing like learning on the job! In the end, it was one of the most rewarding opportunities that I had ever had. The project was completed on time, within one percent of budget and completely operational. To God be the glory!

My Dad

The year was 1979. My mother and dad had moved to Sundridge, Ontario, six years earlier. My dad had always loved the north, and besides, there were other reasons to be there. My second youngest brother, Mark, was buried in the Sundridge cemetery; and my older brother, Jim, Liz, and family lived just five miles north in a little town called South River. It was a great community and incredibly beautiful. My parents were involved in a little church called The Mission, located on a hill at the south end of Sundridge. For several years, they conducted a Bible club in their home, and local kids would come regularly to learn of Jesus and His love for them. My mother had an old piano in the family room, and she would play choruses, teaching the kids the words and the music. She and dad would sing along. Dad had a fine voice! Their example was wonderful to these children. Only heaven will reveal the full impact of their effect on those young lives!

In the fall of 1978, my dad became very ill. It was discovered that he was suffering with incurable bone cancer. It was a very difficult winter for them both. Finally, Dad was admitted to hospital in Orillia where he passed away on June 30 of 1979. The family gathered for his funeral. It was a difficult day and time for us all, but it was a celebration too. We knew that Dad was not lost from us forever, because he knew and loved Christ and had given his heart and life to Him. And so, we had and have a hope and a promise that we will see Dad in heaven, because Mom and each of their children have trusted Christ as well. So had several of their grandchildren!

Two instances come to mind as I recall all of this. Bev and I and some of our siblings spent the following week with Mother, just helping her with banking and Dad's clothes and things. Mom and I went to the little bank in town. We needed to open the safety deposit box and retrieve some papers. The entrance to the vault was narrow, and Mom and I moved through it at the same time and momentarily got stuck. Mom broke down and began to cry. I held her until she was calm again, and she told me that the last time she and Dad had come, the same thing had happened to them. The memory was so fresh for her, and it broke her heart! The other thing I recall was that as we were sitting in her living room, she told me of something she had experienced a night or two after Dad had died. She hadn't told anyone at that point, because she felt people would not believe her. She awoke during the night, feeling lonely and brokenhearted, missing Dad so much; and she clearly saw, at the foot of her bed, an angel who comforted her and said, "You will be okay. Jesus is here with you!" I am not sure if these are the exact words she heard, but I do know one thing for sure! I believed her! I'm convinced that our amazing God sent her that angel that night. These memories are still so fresh in my mind!

Throughout the next two to three years, business continued to grow; and the order board at Excello, London, was booked to capacity. Then the industry and business in general seemed to level off and then started to decline. Competition from foreign manufacturers became more of a reality, and it became increasingly more difficult to be profitable. New orders started to become scarce and difficult to come by. Eventually layoffs both in the factory and in the design department took its toll. Finally, in the early 1980s, the decision was made to close down our facility. Many of us who had been with the company and had invested our lives in it were deeply disappointed. Finally, after several months, everyone had left Excello, leaving just myself and one other long-term employee. We were the cleanup people, moving last skids of excess materials and pieces of remaining equipment to the overhead doors for salvage. It was a very disheartening time! Where would I go from here?

Muriel and Bill

As I mentioned earlier, I have two sisters, Muriel and Sylvia. Muriel was married to Bill (which makes three Bills in our family—a brother, a brother-in-law, and a nephew), and Sylvia is married to Freeman!

Muriel and Bill had five children including Debra-Lynn who lived just about thirteen hours. Ruth Ann came first followed by Bill Jr. then Debra-Lynn, Craig and then Alyson. Craig was about four years older than our Stephen, but they were very close to each other. Craig learned to communicate with Stephen using finger spelling and became very proficient at it. When our family visited them, Craig immediately took charge of Stephen; and the two of them, along with Craig's friends, went everywhere together. Craig was probably Stephen's closest friend ever. Craig even took Stephen along when he was dating Jackie, and Jackie didn't seem to mind in the least. They were like three peas in a pod!

Craig was an excellent football player in high school, and after graduation, he received a football scholarship to attend Liberty University in the United States. As he was preparing to attend, the doctors discovered an abnormality in his blood and confirmed that he was suffering from a blood disorder. It was shortly diagnosed as leukemia.

Craig, of course, could not attend Liberty while under treatment and lived about thirteen months before he passed away in 1986. This was just devastating for Muriel and Bill, their kids, Jackie, and, of course, all of our family. Stephen was brokenhearted. His closest friend was gone. Even though Craig was only twenty when he passed away, he left behind a legacy. He, indeed, was a man of integrity. He believed God and trusted Him with all his heart. Craig's life impacted us all and especially Stephen! He certainly encouraged him in his life's journey!

Multipath Communications

It happened that, several years before, I'd met a Scottish fellow, Alex, at Wortley Baptist Church where we attended with our families. Alex and I developed a close friendship over the years, and we shared many business interests and ideas. He and his wife, Mae, became very good friends with Bev and I. Alex was sales manager for a small, privately owned company that dealt in the sales and service of telephone systems and equipment. They sold mainly to small businesses, including manufacturing companies, legal and accounting offices, schools, and other small to medium concerns.

Alex and I often talked about being involved together in some business venture, because we really felt that we would make good partners! Not only did we share the same faith and beliefs, but we also both had a good understanding of the business world. But, boy, we had a lot to learn!

When the announcement came at Excello that they were closing the plant, Alex and I began to talk more seriously. Also, about that time, the owner of Alex's company, Multipath Communications, announced that it was his intention to sell his business.

Here was our opportunity! However, there were many problems, the biggest of which was the asking price of Multipath's owner. He wanted half a million dollars! Alex and I had very little money and no access to anymore! But, somehow, we knew that it was meant to be. We prayed together, on many occasions, for God's leading and His provision in this venture, but we knew that we needed a miracle!

Well, God provided a miracle! In fact, several! First, I received an excellent severance package. Within a few weeks, Alex and I met a couple of Christian business men, Bill and Bernie, who were both involved in several successful business ventures. After many meetings between the four of us over the next several months, Bill and Bernie agreed to partner with us in the purchase and operation of Multipath Communications. They became our business partners and investors, and together we put a business plan to buy Multipath and to manage it successfully. To this day, I am incredibly thankful for Bill, Bernie, and Alex both for their wisdom and guidance. There is no question that God brought then into my life!

This was a brand-new direction for me! At least, Alex had knowledge of the telephone business, I had none! He had extensive experience in sales. My only sales experience was selling shoes and selling honey for my dad. Before we took over the helm of Multipath, the four partners decided that I would assume the role of company president. Alex would assume the position of vice president of sales and marketing. (I told Alex the position suited him because he knew all about vice!) We were a great team. The first year our sales exceeded one and a half million dollars! Including the two of us, we had a total staff of eighteen, including one sales person, secretary, technicians, and installers. It was quite a team. We operated four service vans and two station wagons. The overhead and inventory control and management were difficult challenges, so were the payroll and the cash flow! We sold Toshiba telephone systems and fax machines. This was at the beginning of the fax machine phase and business was good! The first twelve months we did extremely well! Toshiba of Canada set a goal for us to sell a reasonable number of systems and faxes in the first year. If we could meet this goal, our company, Multipath Communications, would win two all-expense paid, week-long trips to Japan. We doubled this goal within the first twelve months and earned four all-expense paid seven-day trips to Japan! So, Bev and I and Bernie and his wife traveled to Tokyo together! It was an amazing adventure! Bev and I will never forget it!

Multipath was one of several local telephone interconnect companies in London, Ontario, and area, and we were in direct competition with Bell Canada. We found we could compete very well with their telephone equipment sales at first. However, Bell became more competitive as time went by, and we often lost sales to them. Multipath policy was to offer our customers a one-year warranty on all new equipment sales and service. Our service and labor costs began to rise. There were other issues as well. Alex and I managed the business for almost three years and had a great time doing that.

As I look back now, there are many things I would do differently. But we both learned a great deal, and I believe God was preparing me for what lay ahead. When I sold my shares to Bill, he paid me full price, even though the business was on a downward slope. I will always be grateful to Bill! Bill, Bernie, and Alex were my mentors for sure, and I believe God put then into my life just at the right time!

Where Do I Go from Here?

After I left Multipath, I joined one of Bill's companies for a few months but found it did not fit. The year was 1988, and I felt at loose ends.

During those years of the Excello closing, and the time at Multipath Communications, our family of three grew and progressed through school. In June of 1986, Stephen graduated from Robarts School and began his first year at Gallaudet University in Washington DC.

Gallaudet is a federally chartered private university for the deaf and hard of hearing. With the financial help of our provincial government, Stephen was able to enroll. Gallaudet was founded in 1864 and really was the first school for the advanced education in the world. ASL and English were used for instruction at Gallaudet. We were so thrilled that Stephen had been accepted there!

Carolyn was a "first rate" student. She finished grade eight at Westmount Public School with highest honors in 1985 and began Saunders High School in London, graduating in 1990.

Janis began kindergarten at Westmount Public School in 1983 where she thrived! She was a gem, a quick learner! In fact, she picked up finger spelling very quickly; and before we knew it, she could talk with her brother. What a help she and Carolyn were to their mom regarding Stephen. It was amazing. There is no doubt that our girls were God's special gifts to Bev and me!

I met Ross when we served together on the board of a Christian kid's camp called Camp Canbay. Canbay was a small camp located on the shores of Lake Huron. Our friend, Mark, was full-time director, and he and his family lived near the camp. I served as a board member for a few years, and Ross was the secretary-treasurer. We worked well together. Later, Ross and others encouraged me to take over the role of chairman. The camp was a wonderful place for boys and girls from southwestern Ontario to go and have a good wholesome camping experience. One year, our teenage son, Stephen, was asked by the director to serve as a junior counselor to two profoundly deaf campers who applied to attend. The deaf boys had a wonderful week under Stephen's care!

Niagara

Ross and I became good friends. He knew of my leaving Multipath and the fact that I was unemployed. He also knew of my business background. Ross was a senior administrator with a Canadian wholesale hardware supply company located in London, Ontario. D.H. Howden Company sold materials and products throughout Canada to hardware and lumber stores. They also had exclusive rights for several hardware franchises. It was a large operation!

Ross was a wonderful wise mentor to me. He was my senior by about nine or ten years, and I had great respect for him. He was a solid man of faith, trusting God as I did! As he and I chatted about the future, he suggested that I should consider the sales field as an occupation. He felt I was gifted in that area, that I had the people skills to be successful. In fact, he put me in touch with the vice president of sales at his firm. I had not thought of sales! I wasn't sure, but I met with the vice president and was offered a position as a trainee. I spent six months or so learning the ropes, the procedures and company policies. One day, I was invited into his office and offered a position as sales representative for the Niagara Region. I was to be responsible for more than thirty stores from the Burlington to Hamilton area through to Fort Erie which included the whole Niagara Peninsula. I would be paid commission based on the total net purchases of the Niagara stores. My travel expenses would be covered as well. This meant selling our house in London and locating somewhere in the Niagara area. We had lived in London for seventeen years. Carolyn had recently begun studies at Western University, Janis had just begun grade eight, Bev was working, and Stephen was away at Gallaudet University in Washington DC. Talk about upheaval! As

Bev and I considered this and prayed, we felt strongly that God was directing us in this way. We believed that He had opened this door!

It's fascinating to me the way God works. Many believe that, "Whatever happens, happens"; we just sort of take our best shot and "let the chips fall where they may." "Que sera, sera!" I believe differently, so does Bev and so do our kids! It's matter of knowing and trusting God, I mean really trusting Him! Two scriptures come to mind. One is this, my dad's favorite:

> Trust in the LORD with all thine heart; and lean not unto thine own understanding.
>
> In all thy ways acknowledge him, and he shall direct thy paths. (Proverbs 3:5–6)
>
> The other is:
>
> It is the LORD who goes before you. He will be with you;
>
> He will not leave you or forsake you. Do not fear or be dismayed. (Deuteronomy 31:8)

Well, life goes on! In the fall of 1990, we traveled to St. Catharines to search for a house. We felt that St. Catharines was central to my sales territory and would be a good place for us to live as a family. My home base would be my office. We found a great home in the north end of the city and near Lake Ontario. In January of 1991, we packed up our accumulation of belongings and picked up Janis from her friend's house. Janis had been adamant that she was not moving. She was going to stay with her friend and her friend's mom. We asked her to pray about it, and by the time we had to move, she was okay with it. But it was a hard and brave decision for her. We were proud of her! Maybe the dog I had promised to buy her had something to do with it as well! Anyway, just before we left, her friend's dog bit Bev on the leg. Not sure if that was a bad omen or not! Carolyn stayed behind at her girlfriend's home. Both Carolyn and her friend, Brenda, attended Western University. It was difficult to leave Carolyn behind. In a way, it seemed like our family was coming apart!

I had been working the Niagara peninsula and Hamilton and Burlington territory since mid-October, so I got to know the hardware and building center owners and dealers. I enjoyed the freedom and independence of the job, and other than a few wintery days of traveling, it went well. My business grew, my total annual sales being around five million dollars. I prepared a report each Friday for my territory supervisor, met regularly with him, and made dealer calls together. He wanted to observe my approach to customers and my people skills. For the next five years, business in my region grew, dealer relations improved, and overall, things went reasonably well.

We became established in St. Catharines and loved the area, especially Niagara-on-the-Lake, old town. It thrived in spring, summer, and fall, with visitors from all over the world coming to this well-known town with its peach festival and live theater and horse-drawn buggies. There are many attractions. We often loved to go and walk down the main street and visit the unique shops and bakeries and eating places. Surrounding the town are miles of fields of grapes and fruit of many kinds. There are a great number of wineries and bed and breakfasts places and fancy hotels. It's like a "dreamworld" to many.

We found a little church soon after we arrived. Bev was pleased to meet up again a couple of friends, girls she'd grown up with in Windsor. They had moved previously to the Niagara area and attended the same small church. We all became fast friends with them and their families. The congregation had been meeting in a school when we first attended but soon found a building in the north end of the city, and so, less than a year after Bev, Janis and I came to live here in St. Catharines; we'd became a part of Glenridge Bible Church.

We came to love St. Catharines and the area with the lake so close and Niagara Falls just twenty-one kilometers down the road. Winters were not as difficult as in many other Ontario cities. Our snowfall was less, being somewhat protected by the ridge on the Niagara side. Some say we lived in the "Banana Belt" of Canada. I tend to agree!

My job as sales representative for D.H. Howden was interesting and challenging. I loved the contact with people and enjoyed serving our franchise owners and dealers. For the most part, we became good friends. Often, owners would have urgent needs and would contact me, and I would try my best to accommodate them. Sometimes it meant traveling from Fort Erie to Stony Creek or Burlington with a four-gallon can of paint or a construction tool to satisfy a needy customer or even traveling to and from the London warehouse with something a dealer was desperate for. It was called customer service, and it was relationship building!

Carolyn and Indy

Carolyn was doing well at the University of Western Ontario. Her BA was in sociology, and she was a very committed student. Bev and I were so proud of her when she graduated with her degree.

Occasionally, when we talked by phone, Carolyn mentioned her friend, Indy, who was also a student at the University of Western Ontario. Carolyn and Indy had been dating for the last couple of years. Indy's full name is Inderpal Jaswal. Indy and his younger brother were born in Canada. Their parents had moved from India a few years before. Indy's dad worked with the Canadian federal government and his mom worked in early child care.

One weekend they arrived in St. Catharines for a visit. Bev and I were really impressed with Indy and could sense that he and Carolyn cared for each other! In late August of that year, Indy and Carolyn were married. We quickly grew to love Indy! I told him earlier that Bev and I did not have any sons-in-law in our family, only sons and daughters, so when he joined our family, he became our son! God had now blessed us with two sons, Stephen and Indy, and two daughters, Carolyn and Janis. Our family was growing! Carolyn was now working at the Royal Bank.

Janis and Sean

Janis was doing well in high school. She was surrounded by many good friends, but there were seven, including her, that were very close. The seven called themselves the posse and were always together. I often came home late in the afternoon, after traveling with my job, to find three or four or more of them in Janis' room working on their homework (I think). Anyway, they were together! Once, while calling on a major dealer in another city, I was asked if I knew of anyone who would like a little dog, a Shih Tzu whose name was Tippy. I suddenly remembered my promise to Janis, trying to entice her to move with us from London to St. Catharines. Sight unseen, I agreed to take the dog for my daughter. I also did not have Bev's permission! Sometimes, "a guy's got to do what a guy's got to do!" I arrived back at the dealer's office the next day and picked up the dog, cage, bed, food, leash, and everything else. After all, it was a free package deal. Tippy was a cute little black and white thing, and I just knew that Janis would love him. I wasn't so sure about my wife! I traveled back home, the thirty or so miles, arriving in late afternoon, tucked the dog under my arm, and ran up the front stairs of our house to Janis' bedroom before Bev could catch me! Janis and her friends were studying after school in the bedroom, and the door was closed. I quietly opened the bedroom door just enough to slip the dog inside and then closed it and waited for the reaction. There was an instantaneous eruption of excited screams, surprise, and joy. Janis tore out of that door and threw her arms around my neck! As I think back and reminisce on this, I remember how I felt. It was pure joy that I was able to give a gift, a very special gift to my daughter! I often wonder when we are surprised with a gift from our Father in heaven and we respond with delight to Him, how does He feel? Or do we just take it for granted and not even acknowledge Him? I fear that often this is true. It took Bev some time to adjust to this new member of our family and also took some time for her to entirely forgive me!

I think it was first year high school that Janis met Sean Enns. Sean was Janis' age, and they soon became good friends. They seemed to have a lot in common and had the same circle of friends. I had never met him until one day he knocked at our door. He was calling to visit Janis, of course. Perhaps I was a little cool, because I remember thinking, what were his intentions? Was this guy Sean planning to steal my daughter? I guess this is just normal thinking for a Dad! After all, she was just a teenager in high school. Fast forward twenty-five years, Sean David Enns is married to Janis and is an amazing father of one son and two daughters. We love Sean like a son because he is our son! I mentioned earlier Bev and I don't have sons-in-law, only sons; and we are incredibly proud of all three, Stephen, Indy, and Sean. Each is a precious gift from a loving God. We wouldn't trade them for the world!

ITP Brampton

I enjoyed my work with D.H. Howden for five years, but then things began to change. The company was concerned about overhead and rising costs and increasing competition. There were twenty-five or so sales reps throughout the country, and it was decided to reduce that staff and expand territories for the salespeople that remained. One day I received a call to meet with a senior manager who gave me my notice. My territory was being combined with several others, and I would no longer be needed. It was the fall of 1995. I was fifty-five years old without a job! I was very disappointed, very discouraged, and felt broken inside and useless. Without Bev at my side, I was not sure what I would have done. But she was there, my encourager! And, of course, the Lord was with me. I knew it to be true! I had experienced His faithfulness, and I just knew He would see me through! If I wanted to prove His faithfulness to me, all I needed to do was look back at my life. Most of this is recorded in this book. This same God who had brought me this far would see me through and provide for me and my family along the way! I knew this in my heart! I just didn't see how! That is the amazing thing about God! If you are struggling now, like I was then, give yourself honestly to Him alone! I guarantee you, from experience, that He can be trusted!

This is what happened! I prayed, and Bev prayed about a job, a good job for me, something with a future! Then, I suddenly became sick. I had violent pains in my abdomen, so painful in fact that I spent the next five days in hospital. It was discovered that I had kidney stones lodged in the ureter lining and they had to be "blasted out"! Here I was, without work and confined to the hospital. Was this God's answer?

Just out of the hospital, I received a call from a Toronto headhunter asking if I would be interested in interviewing for a sales position with a company in Brampton. Somehow my name had come up, and they knew my history. The call came out of the blue! I was amazed! Blown away! I said yes! Arrangements were made for the next week, and I traveled to Brampton to meet with the sales and marketing vice president of ITP (Industrial Thermo Polymers Limited). This company is now called Armacell Canada Inc.

We hit it off well, and I was invited back to meet with the company owners. This meeting went well, and I was offered a position as their Canadian sales representative. Again, a new adventure for me and a new future! It was a long drive from St. Catharines to Brampton and back at night, about an hour and a half each way, but I loved the work and the challenge. Several months into the job, I was given the position of Canadian sales manager.

ITP had been formed by the two owners and family in 1980. They were technically brilliant! ITP was in the plastics business, specializing in extruded polyethylene foam products such as pipe insulation, sealant joint backer rod (for construction water proofing), and "water noodles," one of the greatest inventions for kid's swimming fun. It seems that every family has at least one of these! I sold these products to major retailers across Canada. The products were well accepted, and business grew under their label "Tundra." I learned the extruded plastics business well and began to understand the manufacturing process! The people I worked with and for were most accommodating. Because it was a privately owned enterprise, it was like joining a family. I felt valued and not just a "cog in a wheel." I seemed to fit!

On the Move Again

It soon became evident that we needed to move closer to my work in Brampton. My drive consumed more than three hours each day, and so, we decided to move to Guelph where I had grown up and where I had family. Three of my brothers, Paul, Bill, and Ian, lived in the area as well as my sister, Muriel, and her husband, Bill. We found a suitable house in the south end and so moved there in September 1995. Janis had finished her high school in June and soon moved to Hamilton where she rented an apartment with three of her friends. She worked in Hamilton in a lady's lingerie store where she was soon promoted to "key holder." Later she was transferred to a Cambridge, Ontario, store. Since it was reasonably close to Guelph, she could live with us and commute. That was nice! Of course, Stephen moved with us and was attending the school for the deaf in Milton, Ontario, for some postgraduate courses. Janis and Sean became engaged in December of 1998 and were married the following August. It was a lovely wedding! Three years later, she enrolled in Niagara College for her diploma in early childhood education. Sean had previously graduated from the same college in computer studies. We were proud of them both!

Soon after we moved to Guelph, my first cousin, Lloyd, and his wife, Carol, contacted us and later met with them and others for a Bible study at their home. This study group, including relatives, friends, and neighbors, continued meeting together for several years. Lloyd and Carol became good friends, as well as cousins. Lloyd was a contractor and builder, specializing in new house construction and extensive home and commercial renovations throughout Wellington County. We were able to support each other through some difficult times, especially with the loss of Lloyd's mom, my aunt, Grace, and his sister, Laura, and a tragic accident that took the life of his niece, Anna. Lloyd and Carol are still two of my valued mentors!

I loved the work at ITP! The whole team was supportive including top management. Our sales team included representatives in both Canada and the United States. In the United States, there were two sales managers, one to oversee all retail sales and the other looking after the industrial side. Approximately two years after I started with the company, the US industrial sales manager left to pursue other opportunities. That left that job open! I applied and was given the opportunity to be the replacement. The job was to work with major distributors in most of the fifty states. Many of my customers were suppliers of waterproofing and related construction materials to large building and construction contractors. Our product was sealant joint backer rod made of extruded polyethylene foam. This product was used in expansion joints in buildings including high rises, roadways and highways, airport runways, and many other applications. It was big business! ITP was a member of a national waterproofing and sealant association in the United States. Many of the members of this association were distributors of the backer rod product I represented and sold to them. Often our president and senior managers would attend conventions held by the sealant association. As a member, my wife and I were privileged to go as well. One of the first conventions we attended was in Bermuda. It was to be four days. My boss came to me suggesting that we stay the whole week. Bermuda is a gorgeous place, and we had a wonderful time and holiday. We are so grateful for these memories. We also attended conventions in Nashville and Scottsdale, Arizona. Another convention was in Napa Valley, California. Unfortunately, Bev was not able to attend this one with me because of her work schedule.

More of Indy and Carolyn

Carolyn decided to continue her studies after her degree, and so she and Indy moved to Brampton where she attended Sheridan College working toward a diploma in human resources. At the same time, Indy was offered a position in quality control at ITP. It was great working in the same place with Indy. He progressed well and was soon promoted to manager of quality control. Carolyn graduated with her human resource diploma and began working in that field with a firm in Toronto. We were so proud of her and so was Indy, of course!

Stephen

During his time at Gallaudet University in Washington DC, Stephen had struggles with learning in some areas, and it was discovered that he had a learning disability. Further studies through their genetic counseling suggested that he may have Waardenburg syndrome. Waardenburg syndrome is a rare genetic disorder most often characterized by varying degrees of deafness, pigmentation changes, and premature graying or white hair. By the time Stephen turned twenty, his hair had turned from blond to white. Stephen returned home in 1990 unable to complete his studies. The year before, he had been diagnosed with Tourette's syndrome which had started in his teen years and began medication for this condition. Neither he or we knew of the long-term side effects of this medication nor how his life would change and how his health would severally decline. Meantime, Stephen was anxious to continue his studies; and so in 1999, he was accepted at NTID, National Technical Institute for the Deaf, in Rochester, NY. NITD is part of Rochester Institute of

Technology. Stephen arrived there with high hopes! Unfortunately, his health continued to deteriorate; and in the year 2000, he had to leave school and return home in St. Catharines.

These were difficult years for Stephen and for all of us. Years later, in 2001, he was diagnosed with tardive dystonia by a brilliant neurologist from University Hospital in London, Ontario. This doctor specialized in movement disorders. Tardive dystonia is a form of tardive dyskinesia, which includes involuntary movements that resemble multiple movement disorders. Tardive means "late" to indicate that the condition begins some time after drug exposure.

Stephen's health deteriorated, and over the course of a short time, he'd lost more than forty pounds. He was so disappointed to have to leave NTID and his many deaf friends there. His hopes and dreams were dashed! As his health declined and his walking became more difficult, he was fitted for a wheelchair. But Stephen hung in there. Even though his health was failing, his faith in the Lord remained strong, but he often asked us why God is allowing this to happen to him. We had no answer for him. We only knew that God had a plan and we trusted this with all our hearts and so did he! We did everything we knew to do for Stephen. There were probably hundreds of doctors and medical specialist visits, many different prescribed medications, leg braces, and more. There seemed no end to it. It was exhausting and worrisome for all of us, but especially for Bev. She understood this medical stuff, and I didn't. I'm not sure if Stephen or I could have survived without her. She was certainly our "rock" in all of this, over these many years. I am enormously grateful to God for her, and so is Stephen!

September 11, 2001

The year 2001 was a tragic one for many people, including the Craig family!

In early September of that year, I had arranged a business trip to meet with some key distributors in Florida, first in Jacksonville, then Miami. From there I would fly to Tampa, pick up a rental car, and drive to Sarasota for a meeting with a prospective client on Wednesday, September 12, then return to Clearwater and Tampa for distributor meetings on Thursday. My return flight was scheduled on Air Canada for Friday morning, September 15, from Tampa back to Toronto. This would be a busy week! Little did I know how drastically my plans would change! It was the week of 9/11—a date that would go down in history as one of the most devastating and heartbreaking in recent history! Almost everyone remembers and can recall exactly where they were that tragic week.

I arrived in Jacksonville late Monday morning, met with our distributor that afternoon, and then enjoyed dinner with him and his wife. I remember we had a great deal in common and enjoyed ourselves immensely. Early the next morning, September 11, I boarded Southwest Airlines for my flight to Fort Lauderdale where I would pick up my rental car from Hertz and drive to my meeting in Miami. I was nicely settled in my seat when the pilot came on the PA to give us news that an airplane had just flown into one of the World Trade Center towers in Manhattan. What immediately came to mind was that a small Cessna or Piper Cub had crashed into one of the towers. It was sad news of course. A private pilot had surely lost his life, maybe even two or three. A few minutes later, our pilot came back on the air to say that he'd received news that the crashed airplane had been hijacked. It seemed odd to me why anyone would hijack a small airplane. Our flight arrived at Fort Lauderdale, and everything seemed in order. I picked up my bag and my rental and got on the road to my meeting in Miami. I turned on the car radio and the news was devastating. The US government had closed all airports in the country including the one I'd just left and the one I was to fly out of later that afternoon. I arrived at my meeting destination and found the whole staff huddled around little televisions watching in wonder as they showed again and again not one but two large passenger airplanes flying directly into both Trade Center towers and then them collapsing before our very eyes. It was surreal, unreal, like a bad dream! But it had really happened. Although all of us were shaken and disoriented, we finally got to meet and discuss some business. I left my client wondering how I should proceed. I decided to continue with my rental car, driving across "Alligator Alley" to south west Florida and then north to Sarasota. This was a "many hour," drive but I was up to it. If the conditions had been less tragic, I would have enjoyed it immensely! I am an "adventurer at heart!" I spoke to my wife and family many times through the next few days. They feared for me. No one knew what was happening in the United States or in the world for that matter. But I had a sense of calmness knowing that God Himself was with me and the He would protect and care for me as He always had. You see, His Spirit lives in me! I knew that for sure, and I never doubted it for one minute! Even now, I still know this sixteen years after this tragic event and I eagerly look forward to what God, our Lord and protector, has in store, but I know ultimately what that is!

As I headed toward Sarasota, I learned from the news that the terrorists had taken their flight training in the very city where I was heading. That was a bit of interesting information for me. I arrived in Sarasota, found my motel, and contacted my two nieces, Shelly and Kim, who lived there. We had a great supper together. The next morning, I met with my potential client and then proceeded to Clearwater and then over to Tampa. On Friday morning, I was ready to go home. Airports had since opened across the country, or so I'd heard. The fact was when I arrived at Tampa International Airport in lots of time for my flight and had already returned my car to Hertz, I found the airport in virtual darkness. Hardly anyone was there. It was an eerie feeling. Airports are always bustling with people and activity. Not that day! I found the Air Canada booth, no one was there. I learned from security that international flights were not operational. Well, here was a new challenge. I phoned my boss, Terry, and he said to stay put and wait. The only problem was that I had committed to speak at my friend Bruce's ordination as a pastor in Barrie, Ontario, on Sunday morning, and I did not want to let him down. Not sure how I was going to do that with no way to get home and thirteen hundred and fifty miles away, but I prayed that God would provide a way! I went back to Hertz rental. They had a big black Lincoln Town car that had New York license and needed to be returned to New York state. They would charge me no mileage! I took it. The problem was there was a storm coming off the gulf, the winds were wild, some said it had hurricane strength. I got on the highway anyway with this strong wind at my tail. There was no one else on the road but me and the heavy Lincoln and a bunch of palm branches. I put my foot to the floor and just kept going. My lifeline was my cell phone, and my wife, daughters, sons, and brothers kept calling me to make sure I was alive and breathing! After several hours, I crossed over into Georgia and finally stopped for a couple of hours in the northern part of that state. At my wife's insistence, I stopped at a small motel around one o'clock on Saturday morning and slept for about three hours. I was on the road again by 4:00 a.m. and finally arrived at the Buffalo airport around 5:00 p.m. Somehow Indy had convinced Park 'N Fly at the Toronto airport to release my car, and he and Sean drove it to the Niagara Falls, Rainbow Bridge border. I took a cab from the Buffalo airport to the border, walked across the bridge, and was released by customs, a free man! An amazing adventure! In all of this, who could even question God's provision and protection? For that matter, who could even question His existence? I sure couldn't, and if you are completely honest, neither could you. A lot of people do that! I remember passing a little card to a cashier; I often give these cards out. He said to me, "Is that about God?"

"Yes," I said, "as a matter of fact it is!"

He said to me, "I don't want it!"

I said to him, "What if you're wrong?"

His answer to me was, "I'll deal with it!" I went away wondering how in the world could he deal with it. What guarantees even his next breath or yours for that matter?

Indy and Sean drove me all the way to Guelph where I was reunited with Bev and family. The next morning, Bev and I arrived at the church in Barrie on time to take part in my friend Bruce's ceremony!

The other very difficult date was October 24 of that same year! Our oldest brother, David, had a massive heart attack and instantly passed away. Dave was my "big brother" but much more than that! Even though we lived miles apart, there was a closeness there, for me at least, that I cannot describe even today! As I write this, almost sixteen years later, there is a part in my heart that is broken, a part that has never healed. Dave was my mentor, perhaps you could say my spiritual guide in a way. We had many telephone conversations and too few visits. He loved the Lord with a practical intensity, and his living example for me was extraordinary! In fact, each of my eight brothers, their wives, and my two sisters and their husbands have had a dramatic and wonderful part in my faith journey. Dave and his beautiful wife and partner, Nancy, are no exception. I am and will be eternally grateful to God for each one in my family. I consider each one not just a gift but a valuable treasure. I know that each one committed their life to Christ, and all except three, Dave, Mark, and Muriel's husband, Bill, are still on that life journey. Those three have gone ahead of us and are waiting for our arrival in heaven, where our Savior, the Lord Jesus Christ, reigns. That's our promised destination for all who truly trust Christ as Savior and Lord. Our parents are there too!

Dave's funeral was a celebration! The honorable lieutenant governor of Quebec, Lise Thibault, was in attendance sitting in her wheel chair at the front of the church. Dave had been her military attaché for several years prior to his death. She regarded Dave highly and was deeply affected by his passing. I had the honor of speaking on behalf of our family. The church was packed. I remember looking down at Nancy as she sat with her children. Her loss of her beloved David was so difficult for her, for her children, and for all of us, but Dave left a lasting legacy, a testimony, and a life well lived that impacted us all immensely. Those memories and experiences are still fresh in our hearts. Every one of the three or four hundred attendees on that day had been personally touched by David's life and by Nancy's life as well. The reason his funeral was a celebration was that every believer in Christ who attended knew, without a doubt, that they would see Dave again, when we greet him in heaven one day! We have that full assurance, for sure!

There are many memories of that day, and even though our hearts were broken and raw at losing our brother so suddenly, there were moments of rejoicing and laughter as we were reminded of the good times. Archie and Paul, Dave's close friends, contributed to the celebration, telling stories of university days, when Dave, who was often the instigators, placed a dead cat in the back of an antique leather chair, inside the upholstery of the competing school's library, or the time he "borrowed" the school's mascot, a large bronze bird with outstretched wings, and had his picture taken from the shoulders down. The photograph was published in the local newspaper. Unfortunately, it included David's legs and feet; and the mascot's owner recognized David's shoes and, therefore, knew who the thief was. These were only two of many antics that Dave was a part of. When they told these stories and others, it caused volumes of laughter for all of us. So, the memories of Dave are good!

I loved Dave's sense of humor! I remember telling him it was a bit twisted like mine! Our dad had a great sense of humor. Dad had rhymes that he would repeat to his family, usually at the supper table when we were all there. I still remember them. One was:

> One fine day in the middle of the night
> Two dead men got up to fight
> One blind man to see fair play
> Two dead men to yell "hurrah."
> A paralyzed donkey walking by
> Kicked the blind man in the eye
> And knocked them through a nine-inch wall
> Into a dry ditch and drowned them all

As young boys, we thought this was hilarious and, of course, memorized it word for word. Some things you just never forget! Most of what we learned, growing up, was wholesome and good, especially if it was from our parents.

Emma

On June 16, 2002, Emma was born, just after midnight! It was Father's Day! (Also, Grandfather's Day). Carolyn and Indy had presented Bev and me with our very first grandchild! A little girl, nine pounds and she was perfect (and still is) and beautiful as well! Wow! What an amazing gift! I remember trooping to the hospital in Brampton anxiously awaiting the birth of this little one, wondering boy or girl. (Carolyn remembers we were all asleep in the cafeteria at the time awaiting her caesarian birth). No one knew except the doctor and the Lord, of course, that it was a girl! We were so thrilled! I kept telling people that Bev and I were too young to be grandparents (but really, we weren't)! I called Emma, "Emma Ruth Craig Jaswal", because I wanted to get all her names in there! (I still call her that!) Indy's Mom and Dad were thrilled too! Emma was their first grandchild as well. I think that Sean was the first of the family to see her, except Carolyn and Indy of course!

More Changes and Challenges

The year 2002 at ITP started off well. I thoroughly enjoyed my work with the company and especially with our many distributors south of the border! I'd made significant friends in the industry, relationships that were important and valuable to me. I found that in sales, people buy from people. I knew that the product had to be of good quality and that it must be needed and must fill a need, but sales was more than that. Over the years, I'd learned that quality relationships in business had to include honesty and integrity. To be honestly successful in business, trustworthiness was key! My whole goal in my job was to be a man of integrity. I wanted my employers to see this as well! That was my purpose!

Travel certainly changed after 9/11 with many more restrictions both at border crossings and with the airlines. The economy was also greatly affected because of the tragic events that occurred the previous year. Our own company was forced to make some changes in their sales and marketing. I was affected directly. My position was eliminated, and I was given my notice that fall. Bev, Stephen, and I were still living in Guelph at the time, but I was now without work. This was a very difficult time for me. I did have a position for a few months with a sister company of ITP, but that did not work out, although it did last me through the spring of 2003.

I did not know where to go from here. Where would I find meaningful employment at my age? I was sixty-three years old. I certainly needed a job! Bev and I talked about what to do. She and I both knew that God would provide. We just didn't know how or when, and honestly, there were some anxious moments, but we were convinced that He would show us what to do. At this point though, I didn't have a single lead.

Mission Aviation Fellowship of Canada

My friend, Ron, was CEO of Mission Aviation Fellowship (MAF) of Canada. Ron and I sometimes had lunch together! One day while having lunch at his favorite "western" café in Guelph, Ron mentioned that MAF was considering hiring a "major gifts" fund-raiser. Having been in sales for so many years, he thought I might fit and suggested I apply. I wasn't sure, but he told me to talk to Bev and pray about it. The requirement was for the new major gifts fund-raiser to raise $2.1 million within a years' time. The money was to be used to purchase a new airplane for the MAF mission base in Angola, Africa.

I discussed it with Bev, and we certainly prayed for God to lead us, but there seemed to be giant obstacles in our way. I'd never asked anybody for money in my life that I could remember, except asking my dad for twenty-five cents when I was little. I remember he turned me down because he didn't have a penny himself and his pay day was two weeks away. Dad only got paid once a month! Sure, I'd been in sales for years, but I had a product to sell, something I could hold in my hand and demonstrate it and guarantee it and deliver it. I always swore I could never sell insurance or securities, because the product was invisible.

Besides, never having raised money, I knew nothing about missions, especially MAF. How would I ever last, raising funds for a mission I knew nothing about? All these questions and no real answers. But somehow, inside, there was this still, small voice saying, "Go and apply. There's an opportunity here! See where it leads!" I applied! It's amazing how God works, if you really believe in Him and trust Him with your life. I know this from experience.

As Christians, as believers, I know that we must trust God when He urges us, and we must move forward believing that something good will come of it. I remember an old preacher years ago talking about walls in front of us and how we need to jump over them, to scale them, trusting God all the way! Perhaps that preacher was in my mind as I applied that day. I've said it many times before, "If we really trust God and want to prove that He's faithful, all we need to do is to look back and remember." We realize then that He is indeed trustworthy and that this same God, who has guided us through the challenges and rough spots of the past, will lead us forward. You can count on it for sure!

Well, that was more than fourteen years ago, as I write this. Fourteen incredible years! First of all, my decision to serve with MAF was confirmed to me in a most remarkable way. My initial goal was to raise just over two million dollars for a much-needed aircraft replacement for our program in Angola, Africa. This challenge was overwhelming to me, never having had any experience in fund-raising before.

Just a few months after joining Mission Aviation, I received an amazing letter from a supporter whom I had met with regarding this most urgent need. Included with the letter was a check for $250,000. An additional $250,000 for this airplane replacement was promised in twelve months' time. What a confirmation to me that God Himself was with me in this, and I knew then that He would see me through!

In November of that year, 2003, I was on my way to Africa, to the country of Angola, to experience firsthand the mission field and how we are called to serve the Angolan people who are so needy. This country had been involved in civil war for more than twenty-six years, and that war had ended just two years before my arrival. At the time that I arrived, it was estimated that there were several million unexploded landmines buried along roadways and rail lines and along pathways. These were close to hundreds of the outlying villages where children lived with their families. These buried bombs were left behind by the warring tribes as they retreated. I remember seeing disfigured people, many with missing limbs caused by exploding mines during and after that devastating war. It was a heartbreaking reminder to me of man's inhumanity to man!

I flew with Jeff, MAF's chief pilot for the Angolan program. We flew commercial airline out of New York and, after more than fourteen long hours in the air, arrived in Johannesburg, South Africa. We were met by Mark, MAF program director for South Africa. Mark drove us to our overnight accommodations, stopping first at a large shopping mall on the outskirts of Johannesburg. On the way to the mall, we passed street after street of large homes, all of which were surrounded by concrete and stone walls, perhaps ten or twelve feet high, the tops imbedded with large broken glass pieces and barbed wire stretched across the tops. These were to prevent thieves from reaching and breaking into the homes. It was so different from our comparatively safe cities at home. When we arrived at the shopping mall, we noticed several South Africans just standing in various places throughout the vast parking area. Mark immediately approached the closest fellow, chatted with him briefly, gave him some money, and pointed to our car. We then went into the shopping area. Mark explained that he had arranged for the fellow to keep his eye on our car for us. Apparently, this was standard practice. Without protection like this, our car could easily be broken into and robbed, sometimes by these same self-appointed guards. But if you paid them, you could rest assured that they would be kept safe. Thus, the "law of the jungle!"

The next morning, Jeff and I boarded Angola Airlines for our four-hour trip northwest to Luanda, Angola. Angola is located just south of the vast country of the Democratic Republic of the Congo where MAF also operates and has bases.

I was not at all prepared for what I saw when I disembarked the airplane in Luanda. The aircraft landed on the tarmac reasonably close to the main terminal. A large stairway was wheeled to the exit door of the aircraft, and every passenger trooped down the steel steps and walked with carry-ons in hand to the main doors of the huge terminal. There were mass confusion and armed guards everywhere. These guards were dressed in three distinct types of uniforms. Later, I discovered that there were military police, local or district police plus army. All these stern-looking military people carried AK 47s or assault rifles, both hands on their weapons, looking and searching in all directions as they milled through the crowd. Most of the people, at least it seemed to me, were in total disarray and confused. There didn't seem any order to anything!

Fortunately, our MAF contact person, an Angolan himself, found us and guided us through the throngs of people to his car, which somehow, he'd managed to park close by. Amazingly enough, we were able to retrieve all our checked luggage, loaded it into his Toyota, and got out of there. I was relieved, for sure!

As we exited the parking area, I noticed just across the street a massive pile of garbage, perhaps a city block long and probably three or four stories high. I remember seeing several kids, way on the top, riffling through the refuse looking for discarded food garbage or at least something to eat or take home. They held dirty plastic bags trying desperately to find something to fill them, perhaps for their families. It's a sight I'll never forget, one of many things that I saw on that trip that has stayed in my mind to this day. As we drove slowly along the highway, there were hundreds of people selling all sorts of trinkets and shirts and many other things. They came running up to our vehicle, eagerly holding up their wares, smiling broadly, hoping we would choose them to buy from. It was their living! The car was stifling hot even with the windows wide open. People along the way had little huts and lean-to's, some with open fires, cooking bits of food for themselves and their families, or trying to sell it to the passersby. It reminded me of a colorful midway without the rides! After at least an hour or perhaps it was two, I don't recall exactly, we arrived at our lodging, a MAF visitor's overnight place in the heart of the sprawling capital. We were tired and exhausted and hot!

The next morning, we drove back to the terminal, past the thousands of vendors along the way, through the chaos of the airport with its security and guns and all; and somehow, we found and boarded our airplane for the final leg of the journey to Lubango and to our MAF base. This had certainly been an adventurous and fascinating and somewhat stressful three days for me! Little did I know of what was yet to come before my return to Canadian soil! We were warmly welcomed by Gary and Doreen, program managers for Angola and our hosts for the week. After an interesting drive through Lubango along muddy and boggy streets (it was the beginning of rainy season), we arrived at the Mission Aviation compound, several acres surrounded by a high stone fence, that included missionary homes, a school, and outbuildings. The guard opened the gate and waved us through. This would be home for the next several days!

Garry and Doreen were wonderful hosts and made me feel at home right from the beginning. I have so many memories of my visit to Angola and Botswana and Johannesburg. These experiences impacted me deeply, some of which are so imbedded in my subconscious that I'm sure I will never forget them. They are still fresh in my mind, even today! Garry and Doreen's small house, inside the compound, was located near two other MAF homes and adjacent to other homes and outbuildings including a school and several maintenance and storage structures, all surrounded by a wall and fence. One high, guard-attended gate was the only entrance and exit. Limited electrical power was provided by the government but was only available for a few hours per day. MAF had a large generator on base providing electricity for some hours as well. The compound was large and was guarded and patrolled night and day by a well-armed guard.

It was rainy season in West Africa in November, and the roads, even in the city of Lubango, were muddy and boggy with deep trenches where the heavy rains had scoured deep gouges from the torrential downpours. Often trucks and vehicles would fall partly into these deep grooves and I'd often see half a dozen Angolan men, soaking wet, heaving a vehicle out of the ruts with one guy behind the wheel to steer and to accelerate at the right time. They sure knew what they were doing, experienced over many rainy seasons, I'm sure! It was fascinating to watch them work!

The day after my arrival, Gary drove me in his Toyota four-wheel drive vehicle, to a bakery a few miles from base. We arrived early morning to a colorful scene just outside the bakery building. Perhaps a hundred or more Angolan women were seated on the ground waiting for the doors to open. They were there to buy fresh bread to feed their families and others. They were dressed in reds and yellows and other bright dresses and casual attire. They appeared happy and joyful, looking forward to their fresh breads. Most had huge woven baskets that they would fill to the brim, set them on their heads; and make their way home again; some had miles to go. This was Saturday, bakery day, a celebration of sorts! Traveling back with our purchases, Gary and I approached a little bridge and stream. Ahead I noticed a lady standing in the water some distance away. Being new in Africa and wanting to take as many photos as possible to show the folks back home, I grabbed my camera and attempted to focus on the lady in the stream. Immediately, Gary said, "You may not want to take her picture. She's naked from the waist up!" And he was right! I hadn't noticed! I didn't take the picture. It was interesting to me that the stream was their source of water for bathing, washing clothes, sometimes their washroom, and often a source of drinking water. This was Africa, and it was certainly an experience for me!

As we drove over the little bridge, there was a pump for drinking water, where several women were filling large pots, placing them on their heads, and then walking along the roadside back to their huts. For some, the walk was a long way, sometimes taking an hour or more.

The next day was Sunday, and together we attended the morning service along with a large crowd of locals. The church was a National Evangelical Church in Lubango. People were dressed in colorful garb, children and parents alike! Although the national language is mainly Portuguese, and I couldn't understand any of it, some of the music and melody was familiar to me, and so I sang along in English. No one seemed to mind! It indeed was a joyous time. The singing was boisterous and loud and exuberant but full of melody! What really stood out for me was when twenty or so young men stood up and sang together a Capello. I don't think I have ever heard such a rich worship sound before, voices blending perfectly, and unaccompanied. It was truly magnificent and praiseworthy. If only we could sing like that in our churches in Canada! I'm sure it would bring joy to the heart of God!

Throughout the course of the week, I experienced some things that will never leave me! I believe it was the next morning. Gary, Jeff, and I drove to Lubango's national airport located several miles across town from our compound. The MAF hanger is located off the tarmac some distance from the main terminal. It was constructed some years ago by stacking forty-foot shipping containers, two high, end to end along both sides and the back, making an 80 foot by 80 foot enclosure with a corrugated sheeted steel roof. Doorways had been cut into the containers making them into offices and maintenance and parts rooms. This was home for our Cessna Grand Caravan aircraft when it was not in use or when it required repair and/or regular maintenance. This improvised shelter also provided a workplace for our two Angolans and our Canadian mechanical staff. Also, goods such as clothing, medical supplies and food, etc. were gathered there and made ready to fly to remote villages for needy and starving people desperate for our help.

After carefully weighing and loading the aircraft, Gary and Jeff (both pilots) guided several NGOs and myself to our seats. I was equipped with a headset, so I could hear both the instructions from the ground and the pilot's conversation during takeoff and flight. I was seated directly behind the right seat, where Jeff, the co-pilot, sat. It was really a frontrow seat! Looking down, I observed two or three Russian military fighter jets parked on the tarmac. I was told that they were used by young Russian pilots to practice takeoffs and landings by permission of the new Angolan government. I observed over the week that I was there, the constant screaming of these aircraft as they regularly practiced their maneuvers over the city and countryside. The other thing that was a bit unnerving to me was a skid containing several torpedo-shaped bombs sitting on the tarmac close to the Russian fighter aircraft. Evidently, these were leftovers from Angola's recently ended twenty-six-year civil war. I saw many evidences of this tragedy!

As I traveled, I often wondered why God had allowed me to experience all of this. Even at my age of sixty-three years, I sensed He was shaping me for something more but wasn't sure what. What was His purpose, His ultimate purpose? Perhaps it was to tell my story, but I believe it was more! I know for sure that I want to be His light to the people I encounter, especially to my family, but also to anyone

I meet. I have the privilege of introducing the God of the universe, the God who is my beloved friend, the Savior of all mankind, to you, if you'll only trust Him. That's my purpose and that is my testimony!

We flew through the clouds heading toward a small village more than an hour away. Our purpose was to bring them supplies, food that they desperately needed, and medical materials. We had UN people on board who were coming to help these needy villagers. As we approached the grassy strip for landing, we circled once to assure that there were no boggy places that could cause difficulty in our landing. When Gary was confident, he set a path. As we touched down, a tribesman guiding two oxen along the perimeter lost control of them, and they headed straight for our spinning propeller. Fortunately, he regained control of his oxen team on time and guided them safely to the side. I'm sure it was the sudden noise of the airplane engine that frightened them. I had visions of chopped oxen and a severely damaged aircraft.

As we left the aircraft, Gary called me to the side. Along the outer edges of the landing path, on each side, a row of large rocks had been placed indicating it was safe to land the airplane between the long rows of rocks. As he and I approached one of the rocks, he pointed to a diagonally shaped item protruding from the ground about ten or twelve meters outside the rock line. Gary asked me what I thought it was. I didn't know. He explained it was an unexploded landmine, one of millions that were left behind by retreating forces. I noticed people including several children who were missing limbs as a result of exploding landmines! So many tragedies in this land!

We piled into a dated jeep of some sort, to travel to the village. The old vehicle was driven by a kindly old nun, much older than the vehicle. I believe she was Portuguese, so we could only communicate with nods and smiles. The people at the small medical clinic were anxious for us to come and visit their little hospital. They were so pleased to receive the supplies. Very seldom did anyone come, especially white people from Canada! It was a dreary day, overcast and damp. It had rained off and on. We entered this little clinic; it was very dark inside. There was no light, except from a couple of small windows, but no electricity. I noticed two things right away, the sound of clicking and a row of four or five black men dressed in sparkling white medical coats, proudly standing in a straight line, almost at attention, just inside the hospital door. These men were so pleased and proud. None were doctors or nurses or were they even paid. They were just volunteers, with hearts of gold! I remember this so clearly! As I peered into the darkness, I found where the clicking was coming from. An aged black lady was sitting at an old typewriter recording patient's medical notes on a paper. How she could even see in the darkness was amazing to me! The young men welcomed us with sincere smiles and handshakes. We had made their day. They toured us through the three or four small rooms, all with mud floors, proudly pointing out their pharmacy with its virtually empty shelves, only containing a few bandages and perhaps one or two bottles of something. I, along with the others, entered a little room on the right. It contained four white, rusty beds each with a small, perhaps one-inch diameter stick tied with a rag to one of the uprights. The stick had a V-shape or short branch, perhaps four or five inches long at the top end. These were to be used as IV hangers, if there was any IV available of course! On each bed sat a young mother breast-feeding her infant baby, perhaps one or two days old. The mothers themselves were doubtfully more that thirteen or fourteen years old. I looked into their faces, and there seemed to be no hope there, only blank stares and despair. I'm not sure their condition nor even if any survived. It seemed so hopeless. We were there to bring them hope and light. *How, Lord?* I cannot get their faces out of my mind. I don't think I ever will! Just inside the door, on the right, sat a woman tending a little fire, cooking something for her half-naked child, possibly two years old or less, who stood close by her, watching us with big round eyes. We were intruders! The good news was that a slightly newer, hospital was being built not far away that could have limited electricity, but I seem to remember that construction was on hold due to lack of materials. There is so much need in Angola, even these many years later.

On the flight back to our base in Lubango, we encountered several dark storm clouds and flashes of lightning. It was amazing to watch Gary maneuver around these flashes and, at the same time, always on the lookout for other aircraft in the area. Ground support was limited at best, and so we had to be especially alert. Our MAF pilots are so skilled, each one specially trained for any challenge.

A few days later, Doreen and another MAF lady missionary accompanied me to a medical clinic in the interior, very remote and several miles from our compound. This little hospital was much more up to date than the one I had visited a couple of days before. It was overseen by a Canadian lady doctor who was indeed a gem! She had managed the clinic for many years. I believe she had tragically lost her husband in an accident just few years before our visit. She lived in a small house close to the clinic, a house surrounded by a high fence with protective barbed wire strung across the top. There was always the fear of thieves and marauders, especially during the night.

Adjacent to the clinic was a small group of huts, about three or four on each side of a wide mud path with a dozen or so small children running and playing between the huts. Their parents stayed in the little huts, most very ill with AIDS or TB or other diseases that were communicable and often fatal. When the children saw me, they clustered around. They were happy and full of fun. I showed them my camera, taking pictures of them and then showing them what they looked like. They were thrilled, running all around me with their bare feet covered with dirt and their tattered clothing. I wondered what their future would be!

We toured the clinic. It was much more up to date than the other but so far below our Canadian standards. At least they had a doctor who loved her patients. That was most evident. She had a very limited amount of medication, but she had the knowledge and experience to analyze and prescribe the cure or at least something to ease the discomfort of these people who came to her for help. Coming out of the far door of the clinic, I almost ran into a very tall thin black man; he may have been seven feet tall, wearing tribal clothing and very scary. An older woman, also dressed in native attire, was stooped over cooking something on a small fire, likely their noon meal. They did not pay any attention to me. He just stood there near me, very straight and very dangerous looking. I moved past them before the series of little huts. The missionary doctor and the other missionaries came behind. The doctor explained that this was a normal occurrence. Often natives would suddenly appear from the surrounding jungle for medical help or treatment of some kind. I followed her to the small huts. She wanted to introduce me to the seriously ill patients in the eight huts. These little one-room shacks were without doors but included a small stoop or step at each entrance. She called each one by name in Portuguese and told them this white man was a missionary from Canada and had come to visit them. Of course, I understood none of this but held each hand and looked into their faces and their eyes. They were so thrilled to think that I had come from so far, to meet them. I believe it was as thrilling for me as it was for them. In that moment, I had brought them joy and something indescribable spoke to me in my spirit, something so deep, I can't explain. I'm not sure I'll ever be able to. If this was my only purpose for coming to Africa, then it was worth everything.

Later that week, I met Dr. Stephen Foster. At that time, he was building a forty-bed private hospital near Lubango. A Canadian surgeon raised in Africa by missionary parents, Dr. Foster, has served over thirty-five years in medical ministries throughout Angola and this hospital, CEML (Centro Evangélico de Medicina do Lubango), has been operating since early 2005.

Today MAF has three airplanes in Lubango flying medical teams from CEML hospital into many jungle villages to perform emergency surgeries and do countless medivac flights. I had the privilege of meeting with Stephen, his wife, and sister along with a dozen or so other folks for a Bible study and prayer time. I was so welcomed and felt so at home. Together, God was allowing us to make a difference in the lives of people for eternity!

Jeff and I also made a side trip to Botswana to encourage our missionary families there. Botswana is located south and east of Angola, almost directly south of Zambia. We stayed overnight at a MAF visitor house. It was very hot and full of mosquitos. I remember opening my small suitcase in the morning (I had not zipped it closed) and a cloud of mosquitos rose from the case. Not sure why they had decided to make their home in there. Maybe just because it was dark! It was a great visit with our people and a good chance for me to meet them.

There were many other experiences during my couple of weeks in Africa. One last thing I recall was on my return flight. I was traveling back alone, as my traveling companion, Jeff, had other responsibilities and needed to stay longer. I flew back to Luanda without incident and would then catch a flight to Johannesburg and then my international flight to return to Canada. Arriving at the Luanda airport and obtaining my boarding pass, I sat waiting for boarding. The airport was teeming with armed military personnel. An official-looking military officer approached me and asked me to follow him to a room. He closed the door and asked me if I had any money. I showed him my Canadian funds, but he wanted to know what Angolan currency money I was taking out of the country. I said none, but he seemed suspicious and questioned me further. Finally, he was convinced and let me return to the waiting area. I was told later that he expected me to give him money. Of course, Canadian currency was of no value to him. I'd forgotten that I had packed away several Angolan coins and a few bills to bring back to Stephen (my son). Anyway, he let me go!

I have enjoyed the challenge at MAF, not just learning about the ministry but meeting people from coast to coast who financially and prayerfully support this valuable work. I got to know the Canadian families who served and are serving in more than twenty developing countries in our world. I am amazed to see their dedication, their commitment, to watch them as they "pull up their roots" and move to serve in a third-world country far from their home, with their young families. I remember praying with a young couple with four small girls, just before they left for Madagascar. The ages of their girls were aged four, twins who were about two and a half years old, and a little baby not more than a couple of months. This amazing couple was called by God to serve as missionaries. The dad was a skilled missionary pilot and the mother, a dedicated missionary mom and teacher. These were some of the extraordinary people that I had the privilege of knowing!

My Brother-in-Law, Bill

Muriel's husband, Bill, was more than a brother-in-law to me! He was my brother! Over the years, we did many things together. I remember one time, in the early years, a bunch of us were playing football together. The mistake I made was playing on the opposing team. Bill hiked the ball and hit me dead-on! Now Bill was a big man, close to two 250 pounds. I weighed about one-seventy. If I shut my eyes and think back I can still hear the impact and feel it, at least in my subconscious! We played golf together, Bill, his two sons, and me. I always came last! My score was way higher than any of theirs! They loved to prod me about that, but it was all in good fun. We went on trips together, went fishing together, and other outings as family. We have fond memories of our Christmas together. Bill was extremely kindhearted; he would literally give you "the coat off his back." One time, I remember Bev and I had planned a trip with our family to Disney, but our car broke down. Bill and Muriel lent us their brand-new Ford for the trip. Amazingly kind! Great memories!

Bill suffered with diabetes, and it got increasingly worse. Later he was diagnosed with cancer. He fought valiantly but succumbed to the disease on July 9, 2005, which happened to be my brother Bill's birthday.

These difficult days really tear our family fabricate. They create holes that cannot be filled or repaired. The good news, in fact, the amazing truth is that we will see our loved ones again, those who have truly trusted Christ as Savior! It's a promise that is written in God's love letter to us, the Bible!

Maya

Maya Elizabeth Jaswal was born August 5, 2005, around 7:00 a.m. She weighed seven pounds and six ounces. This time it wasn't Father's Day or even Grandfather's Day, but it was for me! Carolyn had to deliver by C-section again, but this time she was able to hold her newborn in recovery. Another gorgeous granddaughter presented to Mom and me by one of our beautiful daughters and Indy of course! We had the privilege of looking after Emma through all of this! It was amazing! Emma was a little over three at the time, and according to Carolyn, she said to her mom when she first saw Maya, "I didn't think it was going to be a real baby."

When Grandma asked, "What did you think it was going to be?" Emma responded, "Umm . . . maybe a baby elephant!" We are so proud of these girls and thrilled as we see them develop and grow under the careful direction of their parents. They are building a foundation that is solid and strong, one that will stand fast over time and difficulty. It is a foundation based on faith and trust and commitment and, certainly, a love for God Himself!

Jaxson

Jaxson Sean Enns came into the world on July 5, 2006, our first grandson, our only grandson and our favorite grandson, of course! A very handsome lad, I should add. Obviously, Jaxson did not look like his grandfather, at least on the Craig side! He arrived two weeks early at eight fifty-seven in the morning, weighing seven pounds and two ounces, born at West Lincoln Memorial Hospital in Grimsby Ontario. His mother, Janis, had a difficult time both in labor and delivery. (So did his father, Sean, who held up brilliantly!) But the results were worth it all! Grandma and I were in the northern states when Janis went into labor, so we rushed home at full speed to be at Janis and Sean's side. We weren't going to miss this one and ruin a perfect record! We made it without speeding tickets, and Bev was at her side to encourage her during delivery. I was relegated to the waiting room where I was to sit quietly and to consider how old I was getting, with three grandchildren at my tender age!

Georgia

A little less than two years later, on May 26, 2008, Georgia Mackenzie Hope Enns made her appearance at the same Grimsby hospital! She came early in the morning, at two twenty-eight to be exact. Another beautiful granddaughter! Georgia is really a morning person, but that will probably change when she becomes a teenager. We'll have to wait and see! Georgia was granddaughter number three, and all together, that made four grandchildren. I was sure this was some kind of a record until I remembered that my parents had more than twenty-five of them! Georgia was an easier birth than Jaxson, and of course, Grandma was by Janis' side the whole time. Again, I took up my place in the waiting area with Carolyn, anxiously wondering what was going on in the delivery room. Surely, I could do something helpful like boiling water or sleeping! It's always fun naming your kids, but naming Georgia was unique. My first name is George and Janis wanted, somehow, to carry on her dad's name. Thus, Georgia! Her second name came in memory of a special youth leader whom Janis had as a teenager. Mackenzie Campbell (Ken) was a very special person in Janis' life growing up. Ken and his wife, Janice, and their three children were wonderful in our daughter's life, and when Ken died of a brain tumor, it was devastating for Janis and others. Our Janis wanted to carry on that memory and so named her first daughter Mackenzie. The third name, Hope, came from Janis' sister Carolyn. Throughout whole year, Carolyn had the word hope on her mind and in her heart. She passed her thoughts on to her younger sister, Janis, and so, when the time came, Janis was pleased to include Hope in Georgia's name.

Niagara (The Second Time!)

I think it was collusion! Our four grandchildren along with their two mothers felt it was necessary that Grandpa and Grandma and Uncle Stephen move to and live in St. Catharines where we could be close by (and available as babysitters). We, of course, lived in Guelph, Ontario, where MAF head office is located and where I went to work every day when not traveling. So our grandchildren and their parents began to pray for God to arrange this! In May of 2010, it happened! I had turned seventy and was able to arrange with our CEO to work part-time from my new home in the north end of St. Catharines. The family was ecstatic! I hope they still are!

A year and a half prior to our moving, I had been involved with our church pastor in Guelph and another fellow in an intensive men's ministry training project called a triad. The purpose was to challenge men in their spiritual journey to grow in their commitment to Christ. We studied and shared what was called discipleship essentials, learning and applying and living these valuable principles. This period in my life was extremely important to me and has proven so, in these last ten years. Today, I am part of a triad in St. Catharines that is, no doubt, one of the most valuable parts of my life. The fellows who are involved are closer than brothers to me and have certainly helped to shape my life and the ministry that I am a part of. These guys, Barry, Alan, Dennis, Gilles, Jim, Jordan, and before that Indy and Byron, have encouraged me and challenged me and helped me along the way. I'm not sure where I would be today without them. The Bible includes a proverb that says:

> As iron sharpens iron,
> so a friend sharpens a friend. (Proverbs 27:17)

This is certainly true! I am a living proof of this and so are these friends, these brothers!

Just prior to our leaving Guelph, Stephen developed another health challenge. He suddenly suffered a grand mal seizure. This was scary, both for Stephen and for us. The specialists felt that this was caused as a reaction or a side effect from some of the powerful prescription medication that he is on. Later, after our move, he had a second and third seizure and was placed on an additional medication to control them. Since then, he's had one more but none in the last twelve months.

Stephen's potassium levels started dropping about the same time. Tests showed that his adrenal gland was working too hard. Later, his blood pressure started to escalate. After meeting with two new doctors, it was determined there was a benign tumor on one adrenal gland. In December, a year after our move, he had his left gland removed at Juravinski Hospital in Hamilton. Stephen has experienced many medical challenges over the course of his life. It is remarkable how he has come through all these things. He is certainly an encouragement and an example to all of us!

We settled easily in our new home, a condo townhouse in North St. Catharines. We are close to Port Dalhousie, located not far from Lock 1 of the Welland Canal and overlooking Lake Ontario. It's a beautiful spot! This is home!

Charli

On August 26, 2011, Charli Savannah Enns came into the world. Charli, Janis and Sean's second daughter, was grandchild number five and a fourth beautiful granddaughter for Beverley and me. She was also born at the Grimsby hospital, delivered by a midwife. Again, I sat anxiously waiting in the little room provided for grandfathers and family while Grandma was in the delivery room where all the action was taking place. I guess I couldn't have done much anyway, except get in the way. Charli came out at 6:58 p.m. weighing eight pounds and two ounces. Charli was in distress prior to her arrival, with her heart rate up and down. This caused considerable trepidation, so the medical team had to induce Janis. But Bev and faithful Sean were by her side praying for all to go well. And I was in the waiting room having no idea what was going on. Didn't even know if they needed boiling water!

In the end, it all worked out well; and Beverley and I became the very proud grandparents of five perfect grandchildren, four girls and one boy, and there hasn't been any more since!

Bev and I found a church home, Bethany Community Church, which we love, and Stephen attends a deaf church at Calvary Church not far from us. He has made friends with several deaf who attend Calvary. Because Bethany is large with three weekend services, it's more difficult to get to know many of the attendees, but we have been privileged to be part of a care group, five couples, whom we have become very close to as we meet weekly together, in each other's homes. Bev is involved in a couple of ladies' groups, and I serve on the church missions committee.

Bethany is a Missionary Church and is very intentional in serving people whoever and wherever they might be. There is so much need in our world, not just poverty and sickness and hopelessness and many thousands without a future. Our purpose is to bring them hope and help wherever they are. Really, that is our calling, as a missionary church. And so, we reach out, whether it be in St. Catharines or Toronto or El Salvador or Guatemala or wherever. We want to help with their physical needs and bring them the good news, the Gospel. Our purpose and our command is to be the "light" and the "salt" of the earth.

El Salvador

In March of 2013, I traveled with twenty-four others from Bethany Community Church to the country of El Salvador in Central America. For several years, we had been going to this very poor, developing country to build houses for people who never even dreamed of owning a home. These were corrugated steel homes that were well constructed and could provide shelter from the rains and provide security for the families. Each had three rooms, with two windows and a front and rear door, each with locks. After the home was built, a concrete floor and porch were poured. As a team, we would build ten to twelve of these within about three and a half days. We would contract with the local El Salvadorian people ahead of time to build the prefab portions and transport them to the various sites. As we built the home with the men and women of the villages, we would develop relationships and a trust with them. They always love it when we come, bringing clothing and food and medical supplies and toys for the kids. Poverty is everywhere, but there is a happiness and a joy that is often missing from our own country and people.

I remember the second day after we had arrived. I was helping to prepare a site for our first home. I remember it was early morning and very hot, and I was leaning down moving rocks and clearing the site. Something told me to turn around. Standing perhaps ten or twelve feet away was an El Salvadorian man, perhaps late twenties or early thirties. He was standing between two ladies, about his age. What drew me to him was the huge white bandage covering the right side of his face. Something urged me to go over to him, and even though I spoke no Spanish, I stood by him and asked what had happened to his face. Apparently, he spoke a few words of English.

He took the two edges of the bandage at the top and pulled it down to reveal a horrible large raw hole in his cheek. He said, "Cancer, hospital, tomorrow!" I did not know what to say.

I said, "I'm sorry!" Something inside me said that I need to do more, but what? Suddenly, I remembered that I had a new Spanish Bible in my knapsack that I had stowed on the other side of the building site where I was working. I said to the fellow, "Wait, I have something for you!" I hurried to where I had left my backpack and returned a minute later with the Spanish Bible. The fellow's eyes lit up, and a huge smile appeared on his face. I said, "Here, this is for you, for the hospital, tomorrow!"

With a smile from ear to ear, he said, "Thank you! I read."

I looked for one of our leaders who was close by, and when I told her what happened, she immediately said, "Let's you and I go pray for him." We stood and put our arms around this man, standing in the clearing with his friends and many others and prayed that God would protect him and care for him and heal him when he entered the hospital the next day. We never saw this man again, but I know God heard our prayer. I also feel that the many El Salvadorian folks, who had observed that day, were positively affected and challenged.

This trip to El Salvador made a huge impact on me as had my mission trip to Africa many years before. I had seen real poverty and struggles and people living in tumble down huts. There were some living under makeshift tarps or sheets of wood or pieces of corrugated tin. During my first time, there I was shocked and disturbed. I thought about how we live in Canada, how we don't know what real poverty is, and yet we are not happy or content with our circumstances. We complain about taxes and government and our lot in life. We believe we have rights and deserve these rights and more. We don't acknowledge them as privileges, as I believe we should. We just take them and ask for more. Like they were owed to us!

These El Salvadorian people even though they live in abject poverty, often wondering where their next meal would come, appeared settled and at home. Many thoughts rushed through my mind. What I observed was that despite their difficult lives, they seemed content and happy. They loved their families and it showed. They were a community and we, even though outsiders, were accepted with open arms, as friends. These things I will never forget!

The next year, I returned to El Salvador. I wanted to help these people more, somehow! I was thrilled to see that some recognized me from the previous year; it was kind of nice, like coming home, in a way! Again, there were many experiences; I'll just mention a couple. Our plan was to build ten houses again, and I believe there were twenty-five in our team. Some were assigned to entertain the children with games and stories and others were assigned to get to know the families who would receive new homes, so we could learn clothing and shoe sizes of each family member. When the houses were complete, we provided for each family a large barrel of clothing and an equal-sized barrel loaded with food. This would get them started in their new home. The food and clothing were presented to them at the Key Presentation Ceremony on Thursday of that week along with keys to their front and back door. This ceremony was an incredible and joyous time for both the families and us.

The terrain where we were building was very rough. The ground was full of rocks and very hilly. Most times we had to pull down the old lean-tos and shacks to build the new home. Some folks were apprehensive about us removing their place of living. Through our interpreters, we were able to assure them and reassure them that their new home would be ready that day and it would be far better. Some families numbered only a few and others had as many as ten or twelve children and adults living together and sometimes even more! While we were building, a few chickens and dogs ran around the area and an occasional cow and goat.

Karl and I were assigned house number one. We entered the opening to the little lean-to and sat on plastic chairs to chat with the lady through an interpreter. She was having her feet washed and cared for by Jean, one of our team. Jean's husband Ron was outside working on a nearby house. I remember Jean was so tender caring for this lady. Her feet were callused and hard, a result of walking miles to a little market each day to sell vegetables for which she earned about two dollars a day. Her husband had left her some years before. She lived in this little hut with her son, who was about ten, and her mother, the boy's grandmother who stood in the shadows near the back wall. The grandmother appeared frail and seemed very sad. As Jean washed and creamed the boy's mother's feet, we talked with her through our interpreter about sizes of clothes and shoes and about her new home. I remember two things that happened. Her son came in from playing outside, asking if he could have a drink of water. There was a plastic bowl or container near the little window. He went to get his drink but came back to tell his mother that there was a rat swimming in the water. I believe she said that it was okay to drink and that the rat needed water too. This was what the person interpreting told us. About that time, we heard whimpering and crying and realized that it was the grandma standing in the background. Jean and our leader, Val, and I went over to see what was wrong and how we could help. We learned through our interpreter that she was over wrought because she was not able to help provide food for her family. We calmed her a little, put our arms around her, and prayed for her. In the afternoon, I returned to see how she was. She was calm and greeted me with a smile. I was really blessed by that, that God had allowed us to help her and encourage her. I was thrilled.

    The lady got her house that day and, three days later, two huge barrels of clothing and food. She also received her own key, and Karl and I prayed for her and her mom and son as we stood in the hot sun on that Thursday morning. We presented them with a brand new Spanish Bible. I believe she said she would read it and treasure it!

    The other incident I wanted to mention was meeting with Joseline, a beautiful six-year-old girl. Beverley and I had sponsored Joseline through Compassion several years before, and I had the privilege of meeting her, her four-year-old brother, and their mother. I spent the day with them. It was an amazing time. I had brought several gifts, including a doll, some clothes, a backpack, etc. An interpreter from Compassion helped the whole time with the conversation. Joseline's dad could not come because he was in prison. When he learned I was coming, he made a woven wristband for me. Joseline proudly presented it to me, and I wear it to this day. I prayed that he would be released so he could be united with his family—his beautiful girl, her brother, and his wife. We often receive letters from Joseline and, of course, continue to support her monthly.

There are many more memories I have of my trip to El Salvador, things that I will continue to store in my memory and in my heart. These are remarkable things that God, in His amazing favor, has allowed me to be a part of. I am grateful beyond words!

The Last Chapter

Even though I have entitled this The Last Chapter, I believe it is not the final one, at least in my life. Perhaps I may write a sequel someday! But for now, I want to mention a few last things.

What have I learned? What have I learned from writing this book?

1. I have realized that every single person whom God had brought into my life has helped shape me.
2. I am valuable, and God had and has a plan for my life.
3. Beverley and my children, including my two sons-in-law and grandchildren, are my greatest treasures.
4. Our parents, both sides, and our siblings, their spouses, and their children were and are my precious assets.
5. Our many friends are like stars in the sky.
6. Beverley and I are blessed beyond measure and so grateful to our God in heaven who, at this very moment, is preparing a place for us, with Him for eternity!

Francis A. Schaeffer, a well-known author, was a theologian who published at book followed by a Christian cultural and historical documentary film series entitled *How Should We Then Live*. I have never read the book, nor have I seen the film series, but I'm intrigued by the title.

It asks a question that I need to personalize. I need to change it to "How Should I Then Live?" or How Shall I Live from Now On?

I love the scriptures! There is so much to be learned from them. They are the inspired works of real men and women, who lived what is written in their pages.

Moses, the one who, under God's direction and hand, led the children of Israel from Egypt to the promised land, wrote these words in Deuteronomy 8:11–18 (NIV):

> Be careful that you do not forget the Lord your God, failing to observe his commands, his laws and his decrees that I am giving you this day.
>
> Otherwise, when you eat and are satisfied, when you build fine houses and settle down, and when your herds and flocks grow large and your silver and gold increase and all you have is multiplied, then your heart will become proud and you will forget the Lord your God, who brought you out of Egypt, out of the land of slavery.
>
> He led you through the vast and dreadful wilderness, that thirsty and waterless land, with its venomous snakes and scorpions. He brought you water out of hard rock.
>
> He gave you manna to eat in the wilderness, something your ancestors had never known, to humble and test you so that in the end it might go well with you.
>
> You may say to yourself, "My power and the strength of my hands have produced this wealth for me."
>
> But remember the Lord your God, for it is he who gives you the ability to produce wealth, and so confirms his covenant, which he swore to your ancestors, as it is today.
>
> If you ever forget the Lord your God and follow other gods and worship and bow down to them, I testify against you today that you will surely be destroyed.
>
> Like the nations the Lord destroyed before you, so you will be destroyed for not obeying the Lord your God.

You might say this may be true, but it doesn't apply to me, it doesn't apply to life today, certainly not to my life.

Well, most of us don't have herds and flocks. Nor have we traveled through dreadful wildernesses with poisonous snakes and scorpions. I have never drunk water from a rock or eaten manna.

But I have been tested numerous times. My life at times has felt like a wilderness.

In the end, where does your life come from? Where does mine come from? Who really feeds us and clothes us along the way? Who really protects you and me? Honestly, where does your help and my help really come from?

The psalmist said it this way, and I believe it wholeheartedly:

> I lift up my eyes to the mountains—
> where does my help come from?
> My help comes from the Lord,
> the Maker of heaven and earth.
> He will not let your foot slip—
> he who watches over you will not slumber;
> indeed, he who watches over Israel
> will neither slumber nor sleep.
> The Lord watches over you—
> the Lord is your shade at your right hand;
> the sun will not harm you by day,
> nor the moon by night.
> The Lord will keep you from all harm—
> he will watch over your life;
> the Lord will watch over your coming and going
> both now and forevermore.
> (Psalm 121:1–8, NIV)

This is my story, my testimony, to anyone who reads this book. Your life is different, to be sure. No two stories are ever the same, but your destiny can be the same, by simply acknowledging Christ as Savior, realizing and confessing that He died on the cross for you. That, my friend, will be your salvation and your eternity, for sure! I want to end with this song, written years ago by David Phelps and Gloria L. Gaither.

This is my desire and purpose!

I Then Shall Live

I then shall live as one who's been forgiven.
I'll walk with joy to know my debts are paid.
I know my name is clear before my Father;
I am His child and I am not afraid.
So, greatly pardoned, I'll forgive my brother;
The law of love I gladly will obey.
I then shall live as one who's learned compassion.
I've been so loved, that I'll risk loving too.
I know how fear builds walls instead of bridges;
I'll dare to see another's point of view.
And when relationships demand commitment,
Then I'll be there to care and follow through.
Your Kingdom come around and through and in me;
Your power and glory, let them shine through me.
Your Hallowed Name, O may I bear with honor,
And may Your living Kingdom come in me.
The Bread of Life, O may I share with honor,
And may You feed a hungry world through me.
Amen, Amen, Amen.
(David Phelps and Gloria L Gaither)

Dear reader, if I don't see you ever again in this life, will I see you in Heaven? My sincere prayer is that I will! In the end, it is your decision.

Insight

One day at Starbucks, Dick Craig told his "career story" to some of us friends. An underlying theme in his life story stood out. God was working in Dick Craig's life from way back then and clearly all the way through. The truth shouts out.

So now Dick had captured the story on paper; hence, family, friends, and everyone else can grasp that careful involvement.

Dick's story reveals many lessons.

From a distance, we also get an insight. "Many things happen for a reason and a purpose," even when we don't see it at the time. Our heavenly Parent is nurturing us for eternity.

Many readers will have felt God's involvement in their life.

If not, this book may now awaken their awareness.

About the Author

G. Richard (Dick) Craig comes from a successful business background in manufacturing and international sales. For the past fifteen years, he has served with MAF of Canada (MAFC) in development and fund-raising. MAFC is part of worldwide Christian ministry, using more than 135 small aircraft to bring the good news of the Gospel to thousands in our world who are needy, often desperate and without hope.

Married to Beverley for more than fifty-three years, Dick is father to Stephen and daughters Carolyn and Janis. He is grandfather to five "amazing" grandchildren. Dick and wife Beverley reside in St. Catharines, Ontario, Canada. *My Life, Does It Really Matter?* is his first book.

Lightning Source UK Ltd.
Milton Keynes UK
UKHW012001121118
332221UK00001B/60/P